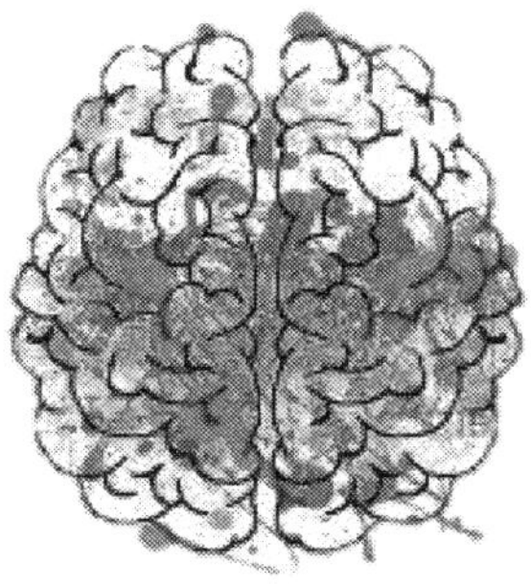

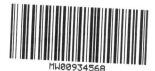

UNMASKING DEMENTIA

"Navigating the uncharted path of memory and identity"

CLAUDE ISAAC

Edited by: Wilcox Samuel and Mark Russo

Design Layout: Joy Margaret

"The disease might hide the person underneath, but there's still a person in there who needs your love and attention." — Jamie Calandriello

TABLE OF CONTENTS

INTRODUCTION

Do you know dementia encompasses a range of disorders characterized by the progressive decline of cognitive abilities? These conditions impair memory, thinking, reasoning, and the ability to perform everyday activities. Understanding dementia involves recognizing its various types, symptoms, and stages of development.

It is a collective term for disorders that affect cognitive function. It typically involves a gradual deterioration in brain function, affecting a person's ability to process information, recall memories, and make decisions. Dementia is not a single disease but a general term that describes a variety of symptoms associated with a decline in memory and other cognitive skills.

Overview of Dementia

Dementia is an umbrella term for a range of neurological conditions that lead to a decline in cognitive function. It affects multiple aspects of mental ability, including memory, thinking, reasoning, and judgment, significantly impairing a person's capacity to perform everyday activities.

Definition and Nature

Dementia is characterized by an irreversible deterioration of cognitive functions. It involves a progressive decline in the brain's ability to function properly, affecting various aspects of daily life. This decline is not a normal part of aging but rather a result of underlying neurological disorders.

Common Features

Progressive Decline: Dementia typically worsens over time, starting with mild cognitive impairment and advancing to severe deficits in memory and reasoning.

Impact on Daily Life: As the condition progresses, individuals may struggle with daily tasks such as managing finances, maintaining personal hygiene, and navigating familiar environments.

Cognitive Domains Affected: Key cognitive functions affected include memory, attention, language, and executive functions (e.g., planning and problem-solving).

Diagnosis and Early Signs

Early diagnosis is crucial for managing dementia effectively. Initial signs might include:

Memory Loss: Difficulty recalling recent events or important information.

Confusion: Disorientation regarding time, place, or identity.

Difficulty with Communication: Trouble finding words or following conversations.

Changes in Behavior: Increased irritability, withdrawal from social activities, or unusual behavior patterns.

Importance of Early Detection

Identifying dementia early allows for better management of symptoms and planning for future care. While there is currently no cure for most types of dementia, early intervention can help mitigate symptoms, provide support for both the individual and their caregivers, and improve the quality of life.

Understanding dementia involves recognizing its impact on cognitive and functional abilities, which helps in providing appropriate care and support to those affected.

Types of Dementia

Dementia encompasses several distinct disorders, each with unique characteristics and causes. Here's an overview of the primary types:

1. Alzheimer's Disease

Description: The most prevalent form of dementia, Alzheimer's disease is characterized by the progressive loss of memory and cognitive functions. It typically starts with mild memory lapses and gradually advances to severe cognitive impairment.

Symptoms: Initial symptoms include short-term memory loss, difficulty in finding words, and disorientation. As the disease progresses, individuals may experience confusion, inability to recognize loved ones, and loss of basic skills.

Pathophysiology: Alzheimer's is associated with the accumulation of amyloid plaques and tau tangles in the brain, leading to neuronal damage and cognitive decline.

2. Vascular Dementia

Description: This type of dementia arises from reduced blood flow to the brain, often due to strokes or other vascular conditions. It can occur suddenly after a stroke or develop gradually as a result of small vessel disease.

Symptoms: Symptoms can include problems with memory, attention, and planning, often accompanied by difficulties in walking and coordination. The pattern of impairment can vary based on the areas of the brain affected.

Pathophysiology: Vascular dementia results from damage to the brain's blood vessels, leading to insufficient oxygen and nutrients reaching brain tissue.

3. Lewy Body Dementia

Description: Lewy Body Dementia (LBD) is characterized by abnormal protein deposits, known as Lewy bodies, in the brain. This type of dementia can cause fluctuations in cognitive function, visual hallucinations, and motor symptoms similar to Parkinson's disease.

Symptoms: Common symptoms include fluctuating attention and alertness, visual hallucinations, and motor difficulties such as tremors and rigidity.

Pathophysiology: Lewy bodies are abnormal clumps of protein that disrupt brain function, affecting cognition, movement, and behavior.

4. Frontotemporal Dementia

Description: Frontotemporal Dementia (FTD) involves progressive damage to the frontal and temporal lobes of the brain, which affects personality, behavior, and language skills.

Symptoms: Individuals may experience significant changes in personality, social conduct, and language abilities. Common behaviors include inappropriate actions, poor judgment, and difficulty in speaking or understanding language.

Pathophysiology: FTD is associated with the degeneration of neurons in the frontal and temporal lobes, leading to distinct patterns of cognitive and behavioral impairment.

5. Mixed Dementia

Description: Mixed Dementia refers to the presence of two or more types of dementia in an individual. Often, this involves a combination of Alzheimer's disease and vascular dementia.

Symptoms: Symptoms can reflect the combination of underlying dementia types, making the presentation more complex and varied.

Pathophysiology: The brain shows pathological features of multiple dementias, such as amyloid plaques and vascular damage.

6. Parkinson's Disease Dementia

Description: Parkinson's Disease Dementia occurs in individuals with Parkinson's disease, a movement disorder that can eventually lead to cognitive decline.

Symptoms: In addition to motor symptoms such as tremors and rigidity, affected individuals may experience memory problems, attention issues, and cognitive decline.

Pathophysiology: The dementia associated with Parkinson's disease is related to the progression of the neurological damage caused by the disease.

7. Creutzfeldt-Jakob Disease

Description: A rare and rapidly progressive form of dementia, Creutzfeldt-Jakob disease (CJD) is caused by abnormal prion proteins in the brain.

Symptoms: Symptoms include rapid cognitive decline, motor dysfunction, and behavioral changes. The disease progresses quickly, leading to severe impairment in a short time.

Pathophysiology: CJD is associated with prion-induced damage to brain tissue, leading to the development of spongiform changes in the brain.

8. Normal Pressure Hydrocephalus

Description: Normal Pressure Hydrocephalus (NPH) is characterized by an accumulation of cerebrospinal fluid in the brain's ventricles, despite normal pressure levels.

Symptoms: Symptoms typically include gait disturbances, urinary incontinence, and cognitive impairment. The condition can often be misdiagnosed due to its overlapping features with other dementias.

Pathophysiology: The accumulation of fluid in the ventricles causes compression of brain tissue, leading to functional impairment.

9. Huntington's Disease Dementia

Description: Huntington's disease is a genetic disorder that leads to progressive neurodegeneration, and dementia can develop as part of the disease's progression.

Symptoms: Individuals with Huntington's disease may experience cognitive decline, motor dysfunction, and psychiatric symptoms such as mood swings and irritability.

Pathophysiology: The disease is caused by genetic mutations that lead to the degeneration of neurons in the brain, particularly affecting the basal ganglia and frontal cortex.

10. Binswanger's Disease

Description: Binswanger's disease is a form of vascular dementia associated with white matter changes in the brain.

Symptoms: Symptoms include memory problems, executive dysfunction, and mood disturbances. The condition often progresses slowly and can be associated with other vascular conditions.

Pathophysiology: It involves damage to the brain's white matter due to chronic ischemia or small vessel disease, affecting cognitive and motor functions.

Each type of dementia presents unique challenges and requires tailored approaches to diagnosis and management. Understanding these differences is essential for providing effective care and support to individuals affected by these conditions.

Understanding Symptoms of Dementia

Recognizing the symptoms of dementia is crucial for early diagnosis and effective management. Symptoms can vary depending on the type of dementia and its stage, but they generally affect cognitive functions and daily living activities. Here's a detailed look at the common symptoms associated with dementia:

1. Memory Impairment

Short-Term Memory Loss: Difficulty recalling recent events, conversations, or newly learned information is often one of the earliest signs. Individuals may forget appointments, repeat questions, or misplace items.

Difficulty in Retaining New Information: Challenges with learning new tasks or absorbing new information can become apparent. This includes struggling to remember recent activities or instructions.

Long-Term Memory Loss: In advanced stages, individuals may also experience problems with long-term memories, such as forgetting significant life events or personal history.

2. Cognitive Challenges

Disorientation: Individuals may become confused about the time, place, or even their own identity. They might get lost in familiar settings or struggle to recognize familiar landmarks.

Difficulty with Problem-Solving: Challenges with planning, organizing, and solving problems are common. This might manifest as difficulty managing finances, following a recipe, or completing a familiar task.

Impaired Judgment: Changes in decision-making abilities can lead to poor judgment or risky behavior. For example, an individual may make unsafe decisions regarding their health or finances.

3. Behavioral Changes

Personality Shifts: Dementia can lead to significant changes in personality, such as increased irritability, aggression, or withdrawal from social interactions. Individuals may become unusually apathetic or exhibit mood swings.

Changes in Routine: There may be a loss of interest in previously enjoyed activities or hobbies. Routine tasks may become challenging, leading to neglect of personal care or daily responsibilities.

Repetitive Behaviors: Some individuals may engage in repetitive actions or behaviors, such as asking the same questions repeatedly or performing the same tasks multiple times.

4. Communication Difficulties

Struggles with Language: Individuals might have trouble finding the right words, following conversations, or understanding complex sentences. This can lead to frequent pauses or incorrect word usage.

Reduced Ability to Express Thoughts: Formulating coherent sentences or expressing thoughts clearly can become increasingly difficult. This can result in fragmented speech or incomplete sentences.

Nonverbal Communication Challenges: Difficulties in interpreting and using nonverbal cues, such as facial expressions or gestures, can also occur. This impacts how well individuals can engage in and understand social interactions.

5. Impaired Executive Functioning

Difficulty Planning and Organizing: Individuals may struggle with tasks that require planning and organization, such as managing schedules, keeping track of appointments, or coordinating activities.

Challenges in Multi-tasking: Handling multiple tasks simultaneously can become overwhelming. Simple tasks may need to be completed one at a time due to decreased ability to manage multiple activities.

Trouble with Abstract Thinking: Understanding abstract concepts or complex ideas can become difficult. This includes problems with grasping abstract relationships or solving problems that require higher-order thinking.

6. Spatial and Visual Difficulties

Difficulty with Spatial Awareness: Individuals may have trouble judging distances, navigating around objects, or understanding spatial relationships. This can lead to issues with mobility and orientation in familiar environments.

Problems with Visual Perception: Visual disturbances, such as difficulty recognizing faces or interpreting visual information, can occur. This includes trouble reading, judging depth, or distinguishing between similar objects.

7. Changes in Behavior and Mood

Apathy and Withdrawal: There may be a noticeable reduction in interest or enthusiasm for activities, leading to social withdrawal and reduced engagement in previously enjoyed activities.

Mood Swings: Rapid or extreme changes in mood, such as sudden outbursts of anger or unexplained sadness, can be prevalent. Emotional responses may become less predictable.

Aggressive or Inappropriate Behavior: Behavioral changes might include aggression, frustration, or engaging in socially inappropriate actions. This can result from confusion, fear, or frustration.

8. Challenges with Daily Living Activities

Difficulty with Personal Care: Maintaining personal hygiene and performing routine self-care tasks can become challenging. Individuals may neglect grooming, bathing, or dressing appropriately.

Problems with Household Tasks: Managing household chores, cooking, and maintaining a clean living space may become overwhelming. Routine tasks may be performed incorrectly or not at all.

Safety Concerns: Ensuring personal safety can become a concern due to impaired judgment and increased vulnerability. This includes issues such as forgetting to turn off the stove or wandering away from home.

Understanding these symptoms helps in providing appropriate care, support, and interventions for individuals with dementia. Early recognition and addressing these symptoms can significantly improve the quality of life and manage the progression of the condition.

GETTING THE DIAGNOSIS

Obtaining a diagnosis for dementia involves a series of steps to ensure accurate identification of the condition. Diagnosis typically includes a comprehensive assessment of medical history, cognitive function, and other relevant factors.

Accurate diagnosis and effective communication are critical for managing dementia. A thorough evaluation, clear discussion of results, and ongoing support help ensure that individuals and their families are well-informed and prepared to address the challenges of the condition.

Seeking a Diagnosis of Dementia

Seeking a diagnosis for dementia is an important step in addressing symptoms and obtaining appropriate care. This process involves recognizing early signs, consulting healthcare professionals, and undergoing comprehensive evaluations. Here's a detailed guide to seeking a diagnosis:

1. Recognizing Symptoms

Early Warning Signs: Pay attention to noticeable changes in memory, thinking, and behavior. Common early symptoms include frequent forgetfulness, confusion about time or place, difficulty performing familiar tasks, and changes in personality or mood.

Monitoring Changes: Track the progression of symptoms over time. Documenting changes in cognitive function and daily activities can provide valuable information to healthcare professionals and help identify patterns.

2. Initial Consultation

Primary Care Visit: Schedule an appointment with a primary care physician (PCP) if you or a loved one notice concerning symptoms. The PCP will conduct an initial assessment to evaluate overall health and cognitive function.

Discussion of Concerns: During the visit, discuss observed symptoms, their duration, and their impact on daily life. Provide detailed information about any changes in behavior, memory, or thinking skills.

Preliminary Testing: The PCP may perform basic cognitive tests and physical examinations to rule out other potential causes of symptoms, such as medication side effects or vitamin deficiencies.

3. Referral to Specialists

Specialist Consultation: If dementia is suspected, the PCP may refer the individual to a specialist, such as a neurologist, geriatrician, or psychiatrist, who has expertise in diagnosing and managing cognitive disorders.

Specialist Evaluation: Specialists will conduct a more comprehensive assessment, including detailed cognitive testing, neuroimaging, and possibly other diagnostic procedures. They will review the medical history, perform a thorough examination, and assess the severity of symptoms.

4. Diagnostic Tests and Procedures

Cognitive Assessments: Standardized tests evaluate various cognitive functions, such as memory, attention, language, and executive skills. These assessments help determine the extent of cognitive impairment and identify specific deficits.

Neuroimaging: Brain imaging techniques, such as MRI (Magnetic Resonance Imaging) or CT (Computed Tomography) scans, provide detailed images of the brain's structure. These scans help identify abnormalities such as atrophy, tumors, or strokes.

Other Tests: Depending on the case, additional tests may include blood tests to rule out other conditions, lumbar punctures to analyze cerebrospinal fluid, or PET (Positron Emission Tomography) scans to assess brain activity and function.

5. Evaluating and Diagnosing

Comprehensive Analysis: Specialists analyze the results of cognitive tests, neuroimaging, and other diagnostic procedures to determine the type of dementia and its severity. They will also consider the individual's medical history and symptom progression.

Differential Diagnosis: It's important to differentiate dementia from other conditions that may present similar symptoms, such as depression, delirium, or other neurological disorders. Accurate diagnosis requires ruling out these conditions.

6. Communicating the Diagnosis

Explanation of Findings: The healthcare provider will discuss the diagnosis with the individual and their family. This includes explaining the type of dementia, its progression, and how it affects cognitive function and daily living.

Discussing Treatment Options: The provider will outline available treatment options, including medications, therapies, and lifestyle changes that may help manage symptoms and improve quality of life.

Providing Resources: Information about support services, caregiver resources, and educational materials will be offered to help navigate the challenges of living with dementia.

7. Planning for the Future

Care Planning: Develop a care plan that addresses the individual's needs and preferences. This may include strategies for managing symptoms, ensuring safety, and making adjustments to daily routines.

Legal and Financial Considerations: Begin discussions about legal and financial planning, including power of attorney, healthcare proxies, and managing finances. Early planning helps ensure that decisions are made in the individual's best interest.

8. Follow-Up Care

Regular Monitoring: Schedule follow-up appointments to monitor the progression of dementia, adjust treatment plans, and address any emerging concerns. Regular evaluations help manage symptoms and adapt care strategies as needed.

Ongoing Support: Continue to seek support from healthcare professionals, support groups, and community resources to address both medical and emotional needs.

Seeking a diagnosis for dementia is a crucial step in managing the condition effectively. By recognizing symptoms early, consulting healthcare professionals, and undergoing comprehensive evaluations, individuals and their families can ensure they receive appropriate care and support.

Understanding the Diagnosis of Dementia

Once a diagnosis of dementia has been made, it is essential to understand its implications, the specific type diagnosed, and the impact it will have on the individual's daily life. Here's an in-depth guide to comprehending the diagnosis:

1. Comprehending the Diagnosis

Explanation of Dementia Type: Understand which type of dementia has been diagnosed (e.g., Alzheimer's disease, vascular dementia, Lewy body dementia). Each type has distinct characteristics, symptoms, and progression patterns. The diagnosis will help determine the most appropriate treatment and management strategies.

Progression of the Disease: Dementia is typically progressive, meaning symptoms will worsen over time. The rate of progression can vary significantly between individuals.

Understanding the expected trajectory of the disease helps in planning and adjusting care as needed.

Impact on Daily Life: Assess how the diagnosis will affect daily activities, including personal care, cognitive functions, and social interactions. This understanding helps in making necessary adaptations to support the individual's needs.

2. Treatment and Management

Treatment Options: Learn about available treatment options, which may include medications, therapies, and lifestyle changes. Treatments aim to manage symptoms, slow progression, and improve quality of life. Understanding the benefits and limitations of each option is crucial.

Medications: Medications may help manage symptoms such as memory loss, agitation, or depression. It's important to be aware of potential side effects and how these medications will fit into the individual's overall care plan.

Therapies: Cognitive therapies, occupational therapy, and speech therapy can assist in managing symptoms and maintaining daily functioning. These therapies are tailored to address specific challenges and improve quality of life.

Lifestyle Adjustments: Incorporating changes in diet, exercise, and daily routines can support overall health and well-being. Adaptations in the home environment may also enhance safety and comfort.

3. Care Planning

Developing a Care Plan: Create a comprehensive care plan that addresses the individual's medical, emotional, and practical needs. This plan should include strategies for managing symptoms, ensuring safety, and supporting daily activities.

Involvement of Family and Caregivers: Engage family members and caregivers in the care planning process. Their involvement is vital for providing support, managing care tasks, and maintaining a stable environment.

Setting Goals and Priorities: Establish clear goals for care, focusing on improving quality of life, maintaining independence as long as possible, and addressing specific needs or preferences of the individual.

4. Support Resources

Educational Materials: Access resources that provide information about the specific type of dementia, its progression, and management strategies. Understanding the condition helps in making informed decisions and coping with its challenges.

Support Groups: Join support groups for individuals with dementia and their families. These groups offer emotional support, practical advice, and opportunities to connect with others facing similar challenges.

Professional Services: Utilize services from healthcare professionals, such as social workers, geriatric care managers, and counselors, who can provide guidance, support, and assistance with navigating the care system.

5. Legal and Financial Planning

Legal Considerations: Address legal matters such as establishing power of attorney, healthcare proxies, and legal directives. These arrangements ensure that decisions can be made in the individual's best interest as their condition progresses.

Financial Management: Plan for the financial aspects of care, including managing expenses, insurance coverage, and budgeting for future needs. Consulting with financial advisors or legal experts can help in making sound financial decisions.

6. Monitoring and Follow-Up

Regular Check-Ups: Schedule regular follow-up appointments with healthcare providers to monitor the progression of the disease, adjust treatment plans, and address any new or emerging issues.

Adjusting Care Plans: Continuously update the care plan based on changes in symptoms, treatment responses, and evolving needs. Flexibility in care planning ensures that the individual's needs are consistently met.

7. Coping with the Diagnosis

Emotional Adjustment: Understand that receiving a dementia diagnosis can be emotionally challenging for both the individual and their family. It's important to address feelings of grief, anxiety, or uncertainty and seek emotional support as needed.

Promoting Well-Being: Focus on maintaining the individual's dignity, respect, and quality of life. Engaging in meaningful activities, fostering social connections, and providing emotional support are key aspects of promoting well-being.

Understanding a dementia diagnosis involves comprehending the specific type of dementia, its progression, and its impact on daily life. It also includes exploring treatment options, developing a care plan, utilizing support resources, and addressing legal and financial considerations. This comprehensive approach ensures that individuals and their families are well-prepared to manage the condition effectively and maintain a high quality of life.

Communicating the Diagnosis of Dementia to the Family

Communicating a dementia diagnosis to family members is a sensitive and crucial step in managing the condition. It involves delivering clear, compassionate information, addressing concerns, and preparing for the future. Here's a comprehensive approach to effectively communicate the diagnosis:

1. Preparation for the Conversation

Gather Information: Before the discussion, ensure you have a thorough understanding of the diagnosis, including the type of dementia, its progression, and treatment options. Be prepared to provide accurate and detailed information.

Choose an Appropriate Setting: Select a quiet, private setting for the conversation. This allows for an open, uninterrupted discussion and provides a comfortable environment for family members to process the information.

2. Delivering the Diagnosis

Use Clear and Simple Language: Avoid medical jargon and use straightforward language to explain the diagnosis. Describe the type of dementia, how it affects the individual, and the expected progression of the disease.

Provide Context: Explain the symptoms and how they relate to the diagnosis. Discuss the impact on daily living, cognitive functions, and overall well-being.

Offer Reassurance: Emphasize that while there is no cure for most types of dementia, there are treatments and strategies to manage symptoms and improve quality of life. Reassure the family that support and resources are available.

3. Addressing Family Concerns

Encourage Questions: Invite family members to ask questions and express their concerns. Provide clear, honest answers and acknowledge that some aspects of the diagnosis may be difficult to understand or accept.

Address Emotional Reactions: Recognize that family members may have a range of emotional responses, including shock, sadness, or anger. Offer support and validate their feelings as they process the information.

Discuss Next Steps: Outline the immediate next steps, including follow-up appointments, treatment options, and any necessary adjustments to the individual's care plan. Ensure that family members understand the plan and their roles in supporting the individual.

4. Providing Support and Resources

Share Educational Materials: Provide resources such as brochures, websites, and books that offer information about the specific type of dementia and its management. This helps family members better understand the condition and how to support the individual.

Recommend Support Groups: Suggest joining support groups for families affected by dementia. These groups offer emotional support, practical advice, and opportunities to connect with others in similar situations.

Offer Referrals to Professionals: Recommend consulting with healthcare professionals, such as social workers, geriatric care managers, or counselors, who can provide additional support and guidance.

5. Planning for the Future

Discuss Care Planning: Begin discussions about developing a comprehensive care plan that addresses the individual's needs, preferences, and safety. Involve family members in the planning process to ensure that everyone is on the same page.

Address Legal and Financial Matters: Talk about the importance of legal and financial planning, including establishing power of attorney, healthcare proxies, and managing finances. Offer resources or referrals for legal and financial advice.

Set Realistic Expectations: Help family members set realistic expectations for the future, including understanding the potential progression of the disease and the impact on caregiving responsibilities.

6. Ongoing Communication

Maintain Open Dialogue: Encourage ongoing communication among family members and with healthcare providers. Regular updates and discussions help ensure that everyone is informed and involved in the care process.

Provide Emotional Support: Offer continued emotional support to family members as they adapt to the diagnosis and its implications. Encourage them to seek counseling or support if needed.

7. Evaluating and Adjusting the Care Plan

Regular Check-Ins: Schedule regular check-ins with family members to review the care plan, address any changes in the individual's condition, and make necessary adjustments.

Adapt as Needed: Be flexible and open to adjusting the care plan based on the individual's evolving needs and preferences, as well as feedback from family members.

Communicating a dementia diagnosis to the family requires sensitivity, clarity, and empathy. By providing accurate information, addressing concerns, and offering support and resources, you can help family members navigate the challenges of dementia and work together to provide the best care for their loved one.

DAILY LIVING WITH DEMENTIA

Managing daily life with dementia involves adapting routines and environments to support the individual's cognitive and functional abilities. It's essential to create a stable, supportive environment that promotes independence while ensuring safety and well-being.

Daily living with dementia requires careful planning and adaptation to support the individual's needs while promoting independence and well-being. By creating a safe environment, managing personal care, engaging in meaningful activities, and addressing behavioral changes, caregivers can help improve the quality of life for individuals with dementia and enhance their daily experiences.

Routine and Structure in Daily Living with Dementia

Establishing routine and structure is vital for individuals with dementia, as it provides stability, reduces confusion, and supports overall well-being. A well-organized daily routine helps maintain a sense of normalcy and predictability, which can be reassuring for those experiencing cognitive decline. Here's a detailed guide to creating and maintaining effective routines and structures:

1. Importance of Routine and Structure

Predictability: Consistent routines help reduce anxiety and confusion by providing a predictable environment. Knowing what to expect throughout the day can help individuals with dementia feel more secure and comfortable.

Cognitive Support: Routines aid in cognitive functioning by minimizing the need for frequent decision-making and reducing the cognitive load. Familiar activities and schedules can help maintain cognitive skills and support memory.

Emotional Stability: A structured routine provides emotional stability by creating a sense of order and control. This can help manage stress and improve overall emotional well-being.

2. Establishing a Daily Routine

Consistent Schedule: Create a daily schedule with regular times for waking up, meals, activities, and bedtime. Consistency helps reinforce a sense of time and reduces disorientation.

Balanced Activities: Incorporate a mix of activities into the daily routine, including physical exercise, cognitive stimulation, social interactions, and relaxation. A balanced schedule supports overall health and engagement.

Flexibility: While maintaining consistency is important, allow for some flexibility to accommodate the individual's changing needs or preferences. Adjust the routine as necessary based on their condition and responses.

3. Morning Routine

Start the Day: Begin the day with a consistent morning routine that includes activities such as personal hygiene, dressing, and a nutritious breakfast. A predictable start helps set a positive tone for the day.

Visual Cues: Use visual cues, such as a daily schedule or picture charts, to guide the morning routine. This can help the individual understand and follow the sequence of activities.

4. Meal Times

Regular Meal Schedule: Plan regular times for meals and snacks to maintain a consistent eating pattern. This helps with appetite regulation and provides structure throughout the day.

Meal Preparation: Simplify meal preparation and involve the individual in cooking when possible. Clear, step-by-step instructions or visual aids can assist with meal preparation tasks.

5. Activity Planning

Scheduled Activities: Plan daily activities that align with the individual's interests and abilities. Include activities such as reading, puzzles, gardening, or light exercise. Scheduled activities provide purposeful engagement and cognitive stimulation.

Routine Integration: Integrate activities into the daily routine at specific times to create a sense of structure. For example, schedule a daily walk after lunch or a favorite hobby in the afternoon.

6. Social and Recreational Activities

Social Engagement: Incorporate regular social interactions into the routine, such as family visits, social outings, or participation in community groups. Social engagement supports emotional well-being and provides meaningful connections.

Structured Leisure Time: Schedule leisure activities, such as watching a favorite TV show, listening to music, or engaging in a hobby. Structured leisure time provides relaxation and enjoyment.

7. Evening Routine

Wind Down: Establish a calming evening routine to signal the transition to bedtime. This may include activities such as reading, listening to soothing music, or engaging in a relaxing hobby.

Consistent Bedtime: Maintain a consistent bedtime to promote healthy sleep patterns. Create a bedtime routine that includes activities such as brushing teeth, changing into pajamas, and preparing for sleep.

8. Adapting the Routine

Monitor and Adjust: Regularly assess the effectiveness of the routine and make adjustments as needed. Pay attention to changes in the individual's preferences, abilities, or condition and adapt the routine accordingly.

Involve the Individual: Include the individual in the process of creating and adjusting the routine. Their input and preferences can help ensure that the routine is meaningful and enjoyable.

9. Using Visual and Auditory Cues

Visual Schedules: Use visual schedules, charts, or calendars to outline the daily routine. Visual aids can help the individual understand and follow the sequence of activities.

Auditory Reminders: Implement auditory reminders, such as alarms or timed notifications, to signal transitions between activities. These reminders can support adherence to the routine and provide cues for upcoming tasks.

10. Caregiver Involvement

Consistency in Care: Caregivers should maintain consistency in the routine and provide support as needed. Consistent caregiving practices help reinforce the structure and stability of daily life.

Communication and Support: Communicate regularly with the individual and other caregivers about the routine and any necessary changes. Provide support and encouragement to ensure that the routine is followed effectively.

Creating and maintaining routine and structure is essential for individuals with dementia. By establishing a consistent daily schedule, integrating meaningful activities, and adapting as needed, caregivers can support the individual's cognitive function, emotional well-being, and overall quality of life.

Managing Behavioral Changes in Dementia

Managing behavioral changes in dementia requires a combination of understanding, patience, and effective strategies. Behavioral changes can include agitation, aggression, confusion, and withdrawal, which can be challenging for both the individual and their caregivers. Here's a comprehensive guide to managing these changes:

1. Understanding Behavioral Changes

Common Behaviors: Recognize that behavioral changes are common in dementia and may include agitation, aggression, anxiety, depression, repetitive actions, and sleep disturbances. These behaviors are often a response to the individual's cognitive and emotional challenges.

Underlying Causes: Identify potential underlying causes of behavioral changes, such as pain, discomfort, unmet needs, environmental factors, or changes in routine. Understanding the root cause helps in addressing the behavior effectively.

2. Identifying Triggers

Observation: Pay attention to patterns and triggers that may lead to behavioral changes. Keep a record of when and where behaviors occur, and what preceded them. This can help identify specific triggers, such as noise, overstimulation, or specific events.

Environmental Factors: Assess the environment for potential triggers, such as loud noises, bright lights, or crowded spaces. Modifying the environment to reduce these triggers can help minimize behavioral issues.

3. Implementing Behavioral Strategies

Calm Approach: Approach the individual calmly and gently when addressing behavioral issues. Avoid reacting with frustration or anger, as this can escalate the situation. Use a soothing tone and body language to convey reassurance.

Redirection: Redirect the individual's attention to a different activity or topic if they are becoming agitated or upset. Engaging them in a calming activity or conversation can help shift their focus and reduce distress.

Validation: Validate the individual's feelings and emotions, even if their reactions seem irrational. Acknowledge their experiences and provide comfort, which can help reduce agitation and frustration.

4. Creating a Structured Environment

Consistency: Maintain a consistent daily routine to provide stability and predictability. A well-structured environment reduces confusion and helps manage behavioral changes by creating a sense of order.

Simplified Space: Simplify the living environment to reduce overstimulation and confusion. Remove clutter, use clear labels, and ensure that the space is easy to navigate and comfortable.

5. Managing Agitation and Aggression

Identify Causes: Determine if there are specific causes for agitation or aggression, such as physical discomfort, unmet needs, or frustration. Address these causes directly to alleviate the behavior.

Calming Techniques: Use calming techniques such as gentle touch, soft music, or relaxation exercises. Create a quiet, soothing space where the individual can retreat if they feel overwhelmed.

6. Addressing Repetitive Behaviors

Redirection: Redirect repetitive behaviors by gently guiding the individual to a different activity. Engage them in an activity they enjoy or find meaningful to help shift their focus.

Meaningful Activities: Provide activities that are meaningful and engaging to the individual. Repetitive behaviors may decrease if the person is engaged in tasks that provide satisfaction and purpose.

7. Managing Sleep Disturbances

Sleep Routine: Establish a consistent bedtime routine and maintain regular sleep-wake cycles. Ensure that the sleep environment is comfortable, quiet, and conducive to rest.

Daytime Activity: Encourage physical activity and mental stimulation during the day to promote better sleep at night. Avoid stimulating activities close to bedtime.

8. Seeking Professional Support

Consult Healthcare Providers: If behavioral changes become severe or unmanageable, consult healthcare providers or specialists. They can assess the individual's condition, provide recommendations, and prescribe medications if necessary.

Behavioral Therapy: Consider behavioral therapy or counseling to address specific behavioral issues. Therapists can offer strategies and interventions tailored to the individual's needs.

9. Supporting Caregivers

Self-Care: Caregivers should practice self-care and seek support to manage their own stress and well-being. Stress management techniques and respite care can help caregivers maintain their own health and effectiveness.

Training and Education: Participate in training and educational programs to learn effective strategies for managing behavioral changes. Knowledge and skills can improve caregivers' confidence and ability to handle challenging behaviors.

10. Encouraging Social Interaction

Social Engagement: Facilitate opportunities for social interaction and engagement with family, friends, or community groups. Social connections can provide emotional support and reduce feelings of isolation or frustration.

Meaningful Participation: Involve the individual in activities and events that align with their interests and abilities. Meaningful participation can improve mood and reduce behavioral issues.

Managing behavioral changes in dementia involves understanding the underlying causes, implementing effective strategies, and creating a supportive environment. By addressing triggers, maintaining consistency, and providing appropriate interventions, caregivers can help improve the individual's quality of life and reduce the impact of challenging behaviors.

Ensuring Safety at Home for Individuals with Dementia

Ensuring safety at home for individuals with dementia is crucial to prevent accidents and provide a secure environment where they can live comfortably. Dementia can affect cognitive and physical abilities, increasing the risk of accidents and making it necessary to adapt the living space accordingly. Here's a comprehensive guide to enhancing safety at home:

1. Assessing the Home Environment

Safety Inspection: Conduct a thorough safety inspection of the home to identify potential hazards. This includes evaluating areas such as the kitchen, bathroom, living spaces, and outdoor areas for safety risks.

Feedback from the Individual: Involve the individual in the safety assessment process if possible. Their input can help identify specific concerns or challenges they may have in navigating their environment.

2. Preventing Falls and Mobility Hazards

Remove Clutter: Keep floors clear of clutter, cords, and obstacles that could cause tripping. Ensure walkways are unobstructed and free from loose rugs or uneven surfaces.

Install Handrails and Grab Bars: Install handrails in stairways and grab bars in bathrooms near toilets and in the shower or bathtub. These installations provide support and reduce the risk of falls.

Use Non-Slip Mats: Place non-slip mats or rugs in areas prone to wetness, such as the bathroom and kitchen, to prevent slipping.

3. Kitchen Safety

Secure Appliances: Ensure that kitchen appliances, such as stoves, ovens, and microwaves, are safely secured and not easily accessible if they pose a risk. Consider using appliance locks or automatic shut-off devices.

Safe Storage: Store knives, cleaning supplies, and other hazardous items out of reach or in locked cabinets. Use childproof locks on cabinets if necessary.

Simple Cooking: Simplify cooking tasks by using appliances that are easy to operate and have automatic shut-off features. Pre-prepared meals or easy-to-use cooking devices can reduce the risk of accidents.

4. Bathroom Safety

Non-Slip Surfaces: Install non-slip surfaces in the bathtub, shower, and on bathroom floors to prevent slipping. Consider using bath mats with suction cups to secure them in place.

Adjustable Water Temperature: Set the water heater temperature to a safe level (usually below 120°F or 49°C) to prevent scalding. Install anti-scald devices on faucets and showerheads.

Accessible Toilets: Use raised toilet seats or grab bars to make it easier for the individual to use the toilet safely. Ensure that the bathroom is well-lit and easy to navigate.

5. Bedroom Safety

Safe Bedding: Ensure that the bed is at a comfortable height for getting in and out. Use safety rails if needed, and ensure that bedding is kept neat and free of obstacles.

Night Lights: Install night lights along pathways to the bathroom and other areas to provide illumination during the night and reduce the risk of falls.

Secure Electrical Cords: Keep electrical cords and wires safely secured and out of the way to prevent tripping hazards.

6. Security Measures

Locks and Alarms: Install locks or alarms on doors and windows to prevent wandering or unauthorized exits. Use alarms that alert caregivers if the individual leaves the home.

Identification and Tracking: Equip the individual with identification, such as a medical alert bracelet or GPS tracking device, in case they become lost or disoriented.

Emergency Contacts: Ensure that emergency contact information is readily available and easily accessible. Post important phone numbers near the phone or on a visible board.

7. Fire and Carbon Monoxide Safety

Smoke Detectors: Install smoke detectors on every floor of the home and ensure they are in working order. Test detectors regularly and replace batteries as needed.

Carbon Monoxide Detectors: Install carbon monoxide detectors near sleeping areas and ensure they are functional. Regularly check and maintain these detectors.

Fire Safety Plan: Develop and practice a fire safety plan, including evacuation routes and meeting points. Ensure that all family members and caregivers are familiar with the plan.

8. Medication Management

Secure Medications: Store medications in a secure, locked cabinet or container to prevent accidental ingestion or misuse. Use pill organizers or reminder systems to help manage medication schedules.

Labeling: Clearly label all medications with dosage instructions and keep them in their original containers. Regularly review and update medication lists with healthcare providers.

9. Personal Safety

Emergency Numbers: Ensure that emergency phone numbers are prominently displayed and easily accessible. This includes numbers for emergency services, family members, and caregivers.

Safe Outings: Plan outings and activities that consider the individual's safety and well-being. Use appropriate mobility aids or transportation services to ensure safe travel.

10. Regular Review and Adjustment

Ongoing Assessment: Regularly review and assess the home environment for safety concerns and make adjustments as needed. As the individual's condition changes, adapt the home to meet their evolving needs.

Ensuring safety at home for individuals with dementia involves a proactive approach to identifying and addressing potential hazards. By creating a secure, supportive environment and implementing appropriate safety measures, caregivers can help prevent accidents and enhance the individual's overall quality of life.

MEDICAL MANAGEMENT

Effective medical management is crucial for individuals with dementia to address symptoms, manage co-existing conditions, and improve overall quality of life. This involves a combination of medication management, regular health assessments, and coordination with healthcare professionals.

Medications and Treatments for Dementia

Medications and treatments for dementia are aimed at managing symptoms, slowing disease progression, and improving quality of life. Treatment approaches vary depending on the type of dementia, the individual's symptoms, and their overall health. Here's a comprehensive overview:

1. Cognitive Enhancers

Donepezil (Aricept):

Function: Increases levels of acetylcholine, a neurotransmitter important for memory and learning.

Usage: Often prescribed for Alzheimer's disease, it can help improve or stabilize cognitive function in mild to moderate cases.

Side Effects: Nausea, diarrhea, insomnia, muscle cramps.

Rivastigmine (Exelon):

Function: Enhances levels of acetylcholine by inhibiting its breakdown.

Usage: Used for Alzheimer's disease and Parkinson's disease dementia. Available as a pill or transdermal patch.

Side Effects: Nausea, vomiting, diarrhea, weight loss, dizziness.

Galantamine (Razadyne):

Function: Increases acetylcholine levels and modulates nicotinic receptors.

Usage: Prescribed for mild to moderate Alzheimer's disease.

Side Effects: Nausea, diarrhea, weight loss, muscle cramps.

Memantine (Namenda):

Function: Regulates glutamate activity, which is involved in learning and memory.

Usage: Used for moderate to severe Alzheimer's disease. Can be combined with cognitive enhancers for better efficacy.

Side Effects: Dizziness, headache, constipation, confusion.

2. Antidepressants

Selective Serotonin Reuptake Inhibitors (SSRIs):

Examples: Sertraline (Zoloft), Citalopram (Celexa), Escitalopram (Lexapro).

Function: Increase levels of serotonin, which can help manage symptoms of depression and anxiety.

Usage: Commonly prescribed to address depressive symptoms in individuals with dementia.

Side Effects: Nausea, insomnia, sexual dysfunction, weight gain.

Serotonin-Norepinephrine Reuptake Inhibitors (SNRIs):

Examples: Venlafaxine (Effexor), Duloxetine (Cymbalta).

Function: Increase levels of both serotonin and norepinephrine.

Usage: Used for depression and sometimes for anxiety in dementia.

Side Effects: Nausea, dry mouth, dizziness, fatigue.

3. Antipsychotics

Atypical Antipsychotics:

Examples: Risperidone (Risperdal), Quetiapine (Seroquel), Olanzapine (Zyprexa).

Function: Used to manage severe agitation, aggression, or psychosis.

Usage: Prescribed with caution due to potential side effects and risks, especially in elderly patients.

Side Effects: Weight gain, diabetes risk, sedation, movement disorders.

Typical Antipsychotics:

Examples: Haloperidol (Haldol), Chlorpromazine (Thorazine).

Function: Manage severe agitation or psychotic symptoms.

Usage: Less commonly used due to a higher risk of side effects compared to atypical antipsychotics.

Side Effects: Extrapyramidal symptoms (e.g., tremors), sedation, weight gain.

4. Anxiolytics

Benzodiazepines:

Examples: Lorazepam (Ativan), Diazepam (Valium).

Function: Used to reduce anxiety and agitation.

Usage: Short-term use only due to risks of dependency and sedation.

Side Effects: Drowsiness, dizziness, impaired coordination, risk of falls.

Buspirone:

Function: An alternative to benzodiazepines for managing anxiety without the same risk of dependency.

Usage: Can be used for anxiety in individuals with dementia.

Side Effects: Dizziness, headache, nausea, nervousness.

5. Medications for Behavioral Symptoms

Mood Stabilizers:

Examples: Valproic acid (Depakote), Lamotrigine (Lamictal).

Function: Used to manage mood swings and irritability.

Usage: Prescribed in cases where mood disorders are prominent.

Side Effects: Weight gain, gastrointestinal issues, tremors.

Anticonvulsants:

Examples: Gabapentin (Neurontin), Pregabalin (Lyrica).

Function: Sometimes used for managing behavioral symptoms such as agitation or aggression.

Usage: Prescribed based on individual symptoms and responses.

Side Effects: Drowsiness, dizziness, weight gain.

6. Non-Pharmacological Treatments

Cognitive Therapy:

Function: Engages individuals in activities designed to stimulate cognitive function and memory.

Usage: Can be used alongside medication to improve cognitive function and manage symptoms.

Behavioral Therapy:

Function: Focuses on managing specific behaviors through structured interventions.

Usage: Helps address challenging behaviors such as aggression or agitation.

Occupational Therapy:

Function: Assists with daily living activities and adapts the environment to improve independence.

Usage: Enhances quality of life by promoting engagement in meaningful activities.

7. Lifestyle and Supportive Treatments

Physical Exercise:

Function: Improves overall health, mobility, and mood.

Usage: Regular exercise can help manage symptoms and improve well-being.

Dietary Adjustments:

Function: Ensures proper nutrition and supports overall health.

Usage: A balanced diet can help manage weight, improve cognitive function, and support general health.

Social Engagement:

Function: Reduces feelings of isolation and supports mental health.

Usage: Encouraging social interactions and participation in activities can enhance emotional well-being.

Medications and treatments for dementia are integral to managing the condition and improving quality of life. A multifaceted approach, including pharmacological treatments, non-pharmacological therapies, lifestyle adjustments, and comprehensive care planning, can help address the various aspects of dementia and support individuals and their caregivers.

Managing Other Health Conditions in Dementia Care

Managing other health conditions in individuals with dementia is crucial for maintaining overall health and improving quality of life. Co-existing health conditions can complicate dementia care and require careful coordination to ensure comprehensive management. Here's a detailed guide to addressing and managing other health conditions alongside dementia:

1. Chronic Diseases

Diabetes:

Monitoring: Regularly monitor blood glucose levels to manage diabetes effectively. Implement dietary adjustments and medication management as prescribed by healthcare providers.

Diet and Exercise: Ensure a balanced diet that supports blood sugar control. Encourage physical activity that is safe and appropriate for the individual's condition.

Medication Adherence: Help manage diabetes medications, including insulin or oral hypoglycemics, to ensure adherence and monitor for side effects.

Hypertension:

Blood Pressure Monitoring: Regularly check blood pressure to manage hypertension and reduce risks of cardiovascular events. Use home monitoring devices if needed.

Medication Management: Adhere to antihypertensive medications as prescribed. Adjust medications based on regular blood pressure readings and healthcare provider recommendations.

Lifestyle Modifications: Implement lifestyle changes such as a low-sodium diet, regular physical activity, and stress management to support blood pressure control.

Heart Disease:

Regular Check-Ups: Schedule regular cardiology evaluations to monitor heart health and manage conditions such as coronary artery disease or heart failure.

Medication Adherence: Follow prescribed treatments for heart disease, including medications for blood pressure, cholesterol, and other related conditions.

Lifestyle Adjustments: Promote a heart-healthy lifestyle that includes a balanced diet, regular exercise, and smoking cessation if applicable.

2. Respiratory Conditions

Chronic Obstructive Pulmonary Disease (COPD):

Medication Management: Adhere to prescribed medications, including bronchodilators and inhaled steroids. Monitor for side effects and effectiveness.

Breathing Exercises: Engage in breathing exercises and techniques to improve lung function and manage symptoms. Use devices such as nebulizers or oxygen therapy as prescribed.

Lifestyle Modifications: Avoid smoking and environmental pollutants. Ensure proper ventilation and air quality in the living environment.

Asthma:

Monitoring and Management: Use asthma action plans and medications, including inhalers and corticosteroids, to manage symptoms. Monitor for triggers and adjust treatment as needed.

Environmental Controls: Minimize exposure to asthma triggers such as allergens, smoke, and pollutants. Ensure a clean living environment with appropriate air filtration.

3. Musculoskeletal Conditions

Osteoarthritis:

Pain Management: Use medications and physical therapy to manage pain and improve mobility. Incorporate low-impact exercises that are gentle on the joints.

Assistive Devices: Utilize assistive devices such as braces or walkers to support mobility and reduce joint strain.

Weight Management: Maintain a healthy weight to reduce stress on the joints. Implement dietary and exercise plans to support weight control.

Rheumatoid Arthritis:

Medication Adherence: Follow prescribed treatments, including disease-modifying antirheumatic drugs (DMARDs) and anti-inflammatory medications.

Physical Therapy: Engage in physical therapy to maintain joint function and reduce stiffness.

Lifestyle Adjustments: Implement strategies to manage joint pain and inflammation, such as gentle exercise and hot/cold therapies.

4. Gastrointestinal Conditions

Gastric Ulcers:

Medication Management: Use medications such as proton pump inhibitors or H2 blockers to manage ulcer symptoms and promote healing.

Dietary Adjustments: Avoid irritants such as spicy foods, caffeine, and alcohol. Implement a bland diet to reduce gastrointestinal discomfort.

Regular Monitoring: Schedule follow-up appointments to monitor ulcer healing and address any complications.

Constipation:

Diet and Hydration: Increase fiber intake through fruits, vegetables, and whole grains. Ensure adequate hydration to support regular bowel movements.

Laxatives: Use over-the-counter or prescribed laxatives as needed, following healthcare provider recommendations.

Routine: Establish a regular bowel routine and encourage physical activity to promote digestive health.

5. Infections

Urinary Tract Infections (UTIs):

Monitoring: Watch for signs of UTIs, such as changes in urination patterns, discomfort, or confusion. Seek medical attention promptly if symptoms arise.

Medication Adherence: Follow prescribed antibiotics and complete the full course of treatment. Monitor for side effects or allergic reactions.

Preventive Measures: Implement good hygiene practices and ensure adequate hydration to reduce the risk of UTIs.

Respiratory Infections:

Vaccinations: Ensure vaccinations are up to date, including influenza and pneumonia vaccines, to prevent respiratory infections.

Monitoring Symptoms: Monitor for signs of respiratory infections, such as cough, fever, or shortness of breath. Seek medical evaluation and treatment as needed.

Supportive Care: Provide supportive care, such as rest, hydration, and medications, to manage symptoms and aid recovery.

6. Diabetes Management

Monitoring Blood Sugar Levels: Regularly monitor blood glucose levels to manage diabetes effectively. Use glucometers and continuous glucose monitors as prescribed.

Diet and Lifestyle: Implement a balanced diet that supports glucose control and encourages regular physical activity. Address any dietary restrictions or preferences.

Medication Adherence: Follow prescribed diabetes medications and insulin therapy. Adjust treatment based on regular monitoring and healthcare provider guidance.

Managing other health conditions in individuals with dementia involves a collaborative approach that integrates medical, lifestyle, and supportive interventions. By addressing co-existing conditions effectively, caregivers can enhance overall health, manage symptoms, and improve the individual's quality of life.

Working with Healthcare Providers in Dementia Care

Effective collaboration with healthcare providers is essential in managing dementia and ensuring comprehensive care. It involves coordinating with various professionals, understanding their roles, and integrating their expertise into the care plan. Here's a detailed guide to working effectively with healthcare providers in dementia care:

1. Building a Care Team

Primary Care Provider (PCP):

Role: The PCP coordinates overall health care, manages chronic conditions, and provides referrals to specialists.

Collaboration: Maintain regular visits to address general health concerns and coordinate care with other specialists.

Neurologist:

Role: Specializes in diagnosing and treating neurological conditions, including different types of dementia.

Collaboration: Work closely with the neurologist to manage cognitive symptoms, adjust medications, and track disease progression.

Geriatrician:

Role: Focuses on the health care of elderly individuals, addressing multiple age-related health issues.

Collaboration: Utilize the geriatrician's expertise in managing complex health conditions and coordinating care for older adults.

Psychiatrist:

Role: Provides psychiatric evaluation and treatment for mood disorders, depression, or psychosis associated with dementia.

Collaboration: Engage with the psychiatrist to manage behavioral and psychological symptoms, including medication adjustments.

Occupational Therapist:

Role: Assists with daily living activities and adapts the environment to support independence.

Collaboration: Work with the occupational therapist to implement strategies that enhance the individual's ability to perform daily tasks and improve quality of life.

Physical Therapist:

Role: Focuses on improving mobility, strength, and physical function through exercises and interventions.

Collaboration: Coordinate with the physical therapist to develop and implement exercise programs that support physical health and mobility.

Speech-Language Pathologist:

Role: Provides therapy for speech, language, and communication difficulties.

Collaboration: Engage with the speech-language pathologist to address communication issues and enhance cognitive-linguistic skills.

2. Effective Communication

Clear Information Sharing:

Provide Comprehensive Information: Share relevant details about the individual's health history, symptoms, and changes with healthcare providers.

Ask Questions: Inquire about treatment options, medication side effects, and the rationale behind recommendations to make informed decisions.

Regular Updates:

Update on Progress: Keep healthcare providers informed about changes in symptoms, response to treatment, and any new concerns.

Coordinate Care Plans: Ensure that all providers are aware of and agree on the care plan to avoid conflicts and ensure cohesive management.

Documenting Information:

Record Keeping: Maintain accurate records of medical appointments, treatments, medications, and observations.

Care Plan Documentation: Keep detailed notes on the care plan and share them with healthcare providers to ensure alignment and consistency.

3. Coordinating Care

Integrated Care Plan:

Develop a Comprehensive Plan: Create an integrated care plan that addresses medical, cognitive, and emotional needs, involving input from all relevant providers.

Monitor and Adjust: Regularly review and adjust the care plan based on the individual's progress and feedback from healthcare providers.

Referral Management:

Manage Referrals: Coordinate referrals to specialists and ensure that appointments are scheduled and attended.

Follow-Up: Follow up on specialist recommendations and integrate their input into the overall care plan.

Care Transitions:

Smooth Transitions: Facilitate smooth transitions between different levels of care, such as hospitalizations or long-term care facilities, and ensure continuity of care.

4. Navigating Healthcare Systems

Understanding Insurance:

Coverage and Benefits: Understand the insurance coverage, benefits, and any limitations related to dementia care.

Manage Claims: Assist with managing insurance claims, authorizations, and documentation for treatments and services.

Accessing Resources:

Utilize Support Services: Access available support services, including case managers, social workers, and community resources, to enhance care.

Advocacy: Advocate for the individual's needs within the healthcare system and ensure that they receive appropriate services and support.

5. Addressing Challenges

Conflict Resolution:

Resolve Disagreements: Address any disagreements or conflicts between healthcare providers or between providers and caregivers.

Seek Mediation: If necessary, seek mediation or consultation with a care coordinator to resolve issues and ensure cohesive care.

Managing Stress:

Caregiver Support: Utilize support groups, counseling, and respite care to manage caregiver stress and prevent burnout.

Self-Care: Encourage caregivers to prioritize self-care and seek support to maintain their own well-being.

6. Education and Training

Provider Education:

Stay Informed: Keep healthcare providers updated on any new developments in dementia care and treatments.

Training Opportunities: Participate in training and educational opportunities to enhance understanding of dementia and effective management strategies.

Caregiver Training:

Education Programs: Engage in caregiver training programs to learn about dementia management, caregiving techniques, and coping strategies.

Skill Development: Develop skills in managing daily care needs, communication techniques, and handling challenging behaviors.

7. Advocacy and Empowerment

Patient Advocacy:

Advocate for Needs: Advocate for the individual's needs and preferences in medical decision-making and care planning.

Empower the Individual: Involve the individual in decisions about their care as much as possible, respecting their autonomy and preferences.

Family Involvement:

Involve Family Members: Include family members in care planning and decision-making to ensure that all perspectives are considered.

Provide Support: Offer support and guidance to family members to help them navigate the care process and understand their role in managing dementia.

Working effectively with healthcare providers in dementia care involves building a cohesive care team, maintaining clear communication, coordinating care, navigating healthcare systems, addressing challenges, and advocating for the individual's needs. By fostering collaboration and ensuring comprehensive management, caregivers can enhance the quality of care and support for individuals with dementia.

LEGAL AND FINANCIAL PLANNING

Legal and financial planning is crucial for ensuring that the needs of individuals with dementia are met and that their wishes are respected. This planning helps manage the complexities of care, protect assets, and navigate legal requirements

Effective legal and financial planning is essential for managing dementia care and ensuring that the individual's needs and wishes are met. By addressing legal and financial considerations proactively, families can provide comprehensive care, protect assets, and navigate the complexities of dementia management.

Financial Planning and Budgeting for Dementia Care

Financial planning and budgeting are essential aspects of managing dementia care, ensuring that resources are allocated effectively to meet both immediate and long-term needs. Here's a comprehensive guide to financial planning and budgeting for dementia care:

1. Developing a Financial Plan

Assessing Financial Situation:

Evaluate Assets: Inventory all financial assets, including savings accounts, investments, property, and personal belongings.

Review Liabilities: Identify and assess any liabilities, such as debts, mortgages, or loans.

Income Sources: Document all sources of income, including pensions, Social Security, and any other benefits or sources of revenue.

Creating a Budget:

Income vs. Expenses: Compare total income to expected expenses to determine how funds will be allocated. Include both fixed (e.g., mortgage, utilities) and variable (e.g., groceries, entertainment) expenses.

Prioritize Needs: Identify and prioritize essential expenses such as medical care, housing, and daily living costs.

Adjust for Changes: Anticipate changes in expenses due to the progression of dementia, such as increased need for caregiving services or medical treatments.

Long-Term Financial Planning:

Project Future Costs: Estimate future costs related to dementia care, including potential costs for long-term care facilities or home modifications.

Plan for Inflation: Account for inflation and potential increases in medical and care costs over time.

2. Managing Medical and Care Expenses

Healthcare Costs:

Insurance Coverage: Review health insurance policies to ensure adequate coverage for medical treatments and medications. Check for additional coverage or supplemental insurance options.

Out-of-Pocket Expenses: Budget for out-of-pocket expenses not covered by insurance, including co-pays, deductibles, and non-covered treatments.

Long-Term Care Costs:

Types of Care: Consider different types of care, such as in-home care, assisted living, or nursing home care, and their associated costs.

Funding Options: Explore funding options for long-term care, including long-term care insurance, Medicaid, and personal savings.

Home Modifications:

Accessibility Improvements: Plan and budget for home modifications to improve accessibility and safety, such as installing ramps, grab bars, or stairlifts.

Emergency Preparedness: Include expenses for emergency preparedness, such as medical alert systems or emergency response services.

3. Financial Power of Attorney

Designating an Agent:

Select a Trusted Individual: Choose a reliable person to act as the financial power of attorney (POA) who will manage financial matters if the individual with dementia is unable to do so.

Define Authority: Clearly outline the scope of authority granted to the financial POA, including handling bank accounts, paying bills, and managing investments.

Legal Requirements:

Draft the Document: Work with an attorney to draft a durable power of attorney document that complies with state laws and clearly defines the agent's responsibilities.

Execute the POA: Ensure the document is signed, dated, and, if necessary, notarized or witnessed according to legal requirements.

4. Insurance and Benefits

Health Insurance:

Review Policies: Regularly review health insurance policies to ensure coverage meets the current and anticipated medical needs of the individual.

Consider Supplemental Insurance: Explore supplemental insurance options, such as Medicare Advantage or Medigap policies, to cover additional medical expenses.

Long-Term Care Insurance:

Evaluate Coverage: Assess existing long-term care insurance policies to understand coverage limits, benefits, and exclusions.

Purchase Insurance: If not already in place, consider purchasing long-term care insurance to help cover future care costs.

Government Benefits:

Social Security: Ensure that Social Security benefits are correctly applied for and that any potential benefits related to disability or caregiving are utilized.

Medicaid: Explore Medicaid eligibility and benefits for long-term care, and understand the application process and requirements.

5. Estate and Legacy Planning

Wills and Trusts:

Draft a Will: Create a will to specify how assets should be distributed upon death and appoint an executor to manage the estate.

Establish Trusts: Consider establishing trusts to manage and protect assets, ensuring they are used according to the individual's wishes.

Estate Taxes:

Plan for Taxes: Develop strategies to minimize estate taxes and ensure that estate planning documents address potential tax implications.

Legacy Planning:

Document Wishes: Outline any wishes regarding legacy, charitable donations, and distribution of personal belongings in the estate plan.

Communicate Plans: Discuss legacy plans with family members to ensure understanding and agreement.

6. Budgeting for Caregiving

Caregiver Expenses:

Compensation: If hiring professional caregivers, budget for their fees, including hourly rates or salary, as well as any additional costs for specialized care.

Respite Care: Plan and budget for respite care services to provide temporary relief for primary caregivers.

Family Caregiving:

Support and Training: Include expenses for training and support services for family caregivers, including counseling or educational resources.

Compensation and Benefits: Explore options for compensating family caregivers or accessing benefits and support services.

7. Managing Assets and Investments

Investment Strategy:

Review Portfolio: Regularly review investment portfolios to ensure they align with the individual's financial goals and risk tolerance.

Adjust for Needs: Adjust investment strategies as needed to accommodate changes in financial needs or care requirements.

Asset Protection:

Protect Assets: Implement strategies to protect assets from potential mismanagement or exploitation, including legal protections and secure storage of financial documents.

8. Navigating Financial Challenges

Addressing Shortfalls:

Identify Gaps: Identify any gaps or shortfalls in funding for necessary care and explore options to address them, such as adjusting the budget or seeking additional resources.

Seek Financial Assistance: Explore options for financial assistance or grants for dementia care, including community resources and nonprofit organizations.

Managing Debt:

Handle Debts: Develop a plan to manage and pay off any existing debts, including negotiating with creditors or consolidating loans if necessary.

9. Monitoring and Adjusting Plans

Regular Review:

Monitor Finances: Regularly monitor and review financial plans and budgets to ensure they remain effective and responsive to changing needs.

Adjust as Needed: Make adjustments to the financial plan and budget as circumstances change, such as shifts in income, expenses, or care needs.

Consult Professionals:

Financial Advisors: Work with financial advisors to review and update financial plans, investment strategies, and budgeting approaches.

Legal Counsel: Consult with legal professionals to ensure that estate planning documents and financial strategies remain current and effective.

10. Education and Resources

Financial Literacy:

Educational Resources: Access educational resources to improve financial literacy and understanding of financial planning for dementia care.

Workshops and Seminars: Attend workshops, seminars, or support groups focused on financial planning for caregivers and individuals with dementia.

Community Support:

Local Resources: Explore local community resources and organizations that offer financial planning assistance, support, and guidance for dementia care.

Online Tools: Utilize online tools and calculators to assist with budgeting, financial planning, and expense tracking.

Effective financial planning and budgeting are essential for managing the costs associated with dementia care and ensuring that resources are used efficiently. By developing a comprehensive financial plan, managing medical and care expenses, and addressing legal and financial considerations, caregivers and families can provide appropriate care and support while safeguarding the individual's financial well-being.

Navigating Insurance and Benefits for Dementia Care

Navigating insurance and benefits is crucial for managing the financial aspects of dementia care. It involves understanding various insurance options, benefits available, and how to optimize coverage to meet the individual's needs. Here's a comprehensive guide to navigating insurance and benefits for dementia care:

1. Health Insurance

Types of Health Insurance:

Medicare: A federal health insurance program for individuals aged 65 and older and certain younger people with disabilities. It consists of:

Part A: Covers hospital stays, skilled nursing facility care, hospice, and some home health services.

Part B: Covers outpatient services, doctor visits, and preventive services. It requires a monthly premium.

Part C: Medicare Advantage plans offered by private insurers that include coverage from both Part A and Part B, often with additional benefits.

Part D: Prescription drug coverage, offered through private plans that can be added to Original Medicare.

Medicaid: A state and federal program that provides health coverage for low-income individuals. It covers a range of services, including long-term care, but eligibility and coverage details vary by state.

Private Health Insurance: Purchased through employers or individually. Coverage and benefits can vary widely, so it's important to review policy details.

Coverage Details:

Inpatient vs. Outpatient: Understand what is covered under inpatient (hospital) and outpatient (doctor visits, therapies) settings.

Specialty Care: Check if the insurance covers specialty services, such as neurologists or geriatric care, which are often needed for dementia care.

Preventive Services: Verify coverage for preventive services, including screenings and counseling, which may be beneficial for managing dementia.

Out-of-Pocket Costs:

Premiums: The monthly cost of maintaining health insurance coverage.

Deductibles: The amount paid out-of-pocket before insurance begins to cover expenses.

Copayments and Coinsurance: Costs paid for each service or percentage of costs after meeting the deductible.

Maximum Out-of-Pocket: The maximum amount you will pay in a year for covered services, after which the insurance covers the remaining costs.

2. Long-Term Care Insurance

Types of Long-Term Care Insurance:

Traditional Policies: Provide coverage for long-term care services such as nursing home care, assisted living, and in-home care. They have daily benefit limits and benefit periods.

Hybrid Policies: Combine long-term care insurance with life insurance or an annuity. They offer a death benefit or return of premium if long-term care services are not needed.

State Partnership Programs: Programs that allow individuals to protect assets while qualifying for Medicaid, often through purchasing long-term care insurance.

Coverage Features:

Daily Benefit Amount: The maximum amount the policy pays per day for long-term care services.

Benefit Period: The duration for which the policy will pay benefits, such as 2 years, 5 years, or lifetime.

Elimination Period: The waiting period before benefits begin, often ranging from 30 to 180 days.

Purchasing and Managing Policies:

Eligibility and Enrollment: Determine eligibility requirements and enroll in a policy before the need for long-term care arises.

Review Policy Details: Regularly review policy terms and benefits to ensure they meet current and anticipated care needs.

File Claims: Understand the process for filing claims and ensure all required documentation is submitted.

3. Government Benefits

Social Security:

Eligibility: Benefits are available to individuals aged 62 or older, or younger individuals with qualifying disabilities.

Disability Benefits: Social Security Disability Insurance (SSDI) provides benefits for those who are unable to work due to a disability, including early-onset dementia.

Supplemental Security Income (SSI): Provides financial assistance to individuals with low income and resources, including those with disabilities.

Medicaid:

Eligibility: Based on income and assets, with specific eligibility criteria varying by state. Medicaid often covers long-term care services that Medicare does not.

Coverage: Includes nursing home care, some in-home care, and personal care services. It may also cover some medical and dental expenses.

Application Process: The application process can be complex; seeking assistance from an elder law attorney or Medicaid planner can be beneficial.

Veterans Benefits:

Aid and Attendance: A benefit for veterans or their spouses who require assistance with activities of daily living. It provides additional monthly payments.

Pension Benefits: Provides financial assistance to eligible veterans and their families. The benefit amount depends on the level of need and other factors.

4. Financial Assistance Programs

Nonprofit Organizations:

Local and National Organizations: Many nonprofits provide financial assistance, support services, and resources for individuals with dementia and their families.

Grants and Scholarships: Explore available grants or scholarships for caregiving support, respite care, or medical expenses.

Community Resources:

Local Agencies: Local government agencies and community organizations may offer financial assistance, food programs, or utility assistance.

Support Groups: Connect with support groups for information on available resources and financial assistance options.

5. Managing Insurance Claims and Benefits

Claims Process:

Documentation: Gather and submit all required documentation for insurance claims, including medical records, care plans, and proof of expenses.

Follow-Up: Regularly follow up on the status of claims to ensure timely processing and address any issues or denials.

Appealing Denied Claims:

Understand Reasons: Review denial letters to understand why claims were denied and gather necessary information for appeal.

File an Appeal: Follow the insurance company's appeal process to contest denied claims. Provide additional documentation or clarification as needed.

Navigating insurance and benefits for dementia care involves understanding various types of coverage, optimizing available resources, and planning effectively for both current and future needs. By carefully managing insurance policies, leveraging government benefits, and seeking professional advice, families can ensure that financial resources are used efficiently to support the individual's care and well-being.

CAREGIVING TECHNIQUES

Effective caregiving for individuals with dementia requires a combination of practical techniques and compassionate approaches. These techniques are designed to improve the quality of care, enhance the individual's well-being, and support caregivers in managing daily challenges.

Effective Communication Strategies in Dementia Care

Effective communication is crucial in dementia care to ensure that interactions are clear, supportive, and respectful. As dementia progresses, the ability to communicate may decline, making it essential for caregivers to adapt their strategies. Here's a comprehensive guide to effective communication strategies in dementia care:

1. Simplify Communication

Use Clear and Simple Language:

Short Sentences: Speak in short, simple sentences to make information easier to understand. Avoid complex sentences and jargon.

Direct Statements: Use direct and specific statements rather than vague questions or suggestions. For example, instead of asking "Do you want to go for a walk?" say "Let's go for a walk now."

Give One Instruction at a Time:

Step-by-Step Guidance: Provide one instruction at a time and break tasks into manageable steps. For instance, instead of saying "Get ready for bed," break it down to "First, put on your pajamas."

Use Visual Aids:

Visual Cues: Incorporate visual aids like pictures, labels, or written instructions to support verbal communication. Visuals can help reinforce understanding and memory.

2. Enhance Non-Verbal Communication

Maintain Positive Body Language:

Open Posture: Use open and approachable body language, such as maintaining eye contact and smiling. Avoid crossing arms or appearing distant.

Gentle Touch: Offer gentle touches or hand-holding if appropriate and comforting. Physical touch can convey reassurance and support.

Use Gestures and Facial Expressions:

Demonstrate Actions: Use gestures to demonstrate actions or intentions. For example, mimic brushing teeth if explaining the process.

Express Emotion: Use facial expressions to convey warmth, empathy, and understanding. Positive facial expressions can help create a supportive atmosphere.

Adapt to Individual Preferences:

Personal Comfort: Pay attention to the individual's non-verbal cues and preferences. Some people may respond better to physical proximity or specific gestures.

3. Facilitate Understanding

Verify Understanding:

Ask for Confirmation: Check for understanding by asking the individual to repeat or explain what they heard. For example, "Can you tell me what we're going to do next?"

Clarify Misunderstandings: Gently clarify any misunderstandings without causing frustration. Rephrase or repeat information if necessary.

Be Patient and Allow Time:

Give Time to Respond: Allow ample time for the individual to process information and respond. Avoid rushing or finishing their sentences for them.

Avoid Interruptions: Minimize interruptions and distractions during conversations. Create a calm environment to facilitate effective communication.

Encourage and Support Expression:

Support Verbal and Non-Verbal Communication: Encourage the individual to express themselves in any way they can, whether through words, gestures, or other forms of communication.

Validate Feelings: Acknowledge and validate the individual's emotions and feelings. Show understanding and empathy in response to their expressions.

4. Adapt Communication Techniques

Use Reminiscence and Familiar Topics:

Engage with Memories: Discuss familiar topics or past experiences that may be more accessible and engaging for the individual. Reminiscence can stimulate positive emotions and connection.

Incorporate Interests: Incorporate the individual's interests and hobbies into conversations to maintain engagement and relevance.

Modify Speech Patterns:

Speak Slowly and Clearly: Articulate words slowly and clearly, but avoid speaking in a condescending manner. Use a calm, even tone of voice.

Emphasize Key Points: Emphasize important information through repetition or emphasis. For instance, repeat key points or instructions for clarity.

Utilize Visual and Sensory Stimuli:

Incorporate Visuals: Use visual aids such as pictures, charts, or objects related to the topic of discussion. Visuals can help reinforce understanding and memory.

Engage the Senses: Incorporate sensory stimuli such as familiar scents, sounds, or textures to enhance communication and create a multisensory experience.

5. Address Behavioral Challenges

Recognize and Manage Agitation:

Stay Calm: Remain calm and composed if the individual becomes agitated or upset. Use a soothing tone and gentle gestures to de-escalate the situation.

Redirect Attention: Redirect the individual's attention to a different activity or topic if they become agitated. Offer a calming distraction or change of focus.

Use Positive Reinforcement:

Encourage Positive Behavior: Offer praise and positive reinforcement for desired behaviors and responses. Acknowledge and celebrate small achievements.

Avoid Criticism: Avoid criticizing or correcting the individual harshly. Instead, use positive language and gentle guidance to encourage appropriate behavior.

Provide Reassurance and Comfort:

Offer Reassurance: Provide reassurance and comfort during moments of confusion or distress. Use a soothing tone and calming presence to offer support.

Create a Safe Space: Ensure that the environment is safe and comforting. Address any sources of discomfort or distress that may be contributing to behavioral challenges.

6. Foster Social Engagement

Facilitate Social Interaction:

Encourage Participation: Encourage the individual to participate in social activities and interactions with family and friends. Social engagement can improve mood and reduce feelings of isolation.

Arrange Social Opportunities: Plan and arrange social opportunities such as visits, group activities, or community events to foster social connections.

Respect Personal Preferences:

Honor Choices: Respect the individual's preferences for social interaction. Some may prefer one-on-one interactions or smaller groups, while others may enjoy larger gatherings.

Adapt Activities: Adapt social activities to suit the individual's abilities and interests. Ensure that activities are enjoyable and meaningful to them.

Monitor and Adjust:

Observe Reactions: Monitor the individual's reactions to social interactions and adjust activities as needed. Be attentive to their comfort level and preferences.

Provide Support: Offer support and assistance during social interactions to ensure that the individual feels comfortable and included.

7. Manage Communication Challenges

Address Memory Loss:

Use Reminders: Use memory aids such as reminders, calendars, or notebooks to help the individual remember important information and appointments.

Reinforce Information: Reinforce important information through repetition and visual cues. Ensure that key points are communicated clearly and consistently.

Adapt to Cognitive Decline:

Adjust Expectations: Adjust expectations based on the individual's cognitive abilities. Be patient and flexible in communication approaches.

Simplify Requests: Simplify requests and tasks to match the individual's current cognitive abilities. Offer clear, step-by-step instructions for complex tasks.

Provide Reassurance and Consistency:

Maintain Consistency: Maintain consistent communication patterns and routines to provide stability and reduce confusion.

Reassure and Comfort: Offer reassurance and comfort to alleviate any anxiety or frustration related to communication difficulties.

8. Encourage Participation and Engagement

Involve in Decision-Making:

Empower Choices: Involve the individual in decision-making processes and allow them to make choices when possible. Empowering them to make decisions fosters a sense of autonomy and engagement.

Offer Options: Provide options and choices rather than open-ended questions. For example, offer two choices and let the individual select their preference.

Promote Active Engagement:

Encourage Participation: Encourage active participation in daily activities and conversations. Offer opportunities for the individual to contribute and be involved.

Create Meaningful Experiences: Engage the individual in activities and discussions that are meaningful and relevant to their interests and experiences.

9. Utilize Technological Aids

Assistive Technology:

Use Communication Devices: Utilize assistive communication devices or apps designed to support verbal and non-verbal communication. These tools can enhance communication and interaction.

Implement Memory Aids: Use digital memory aids, such as reminder apps or electronic calendars, to support memory and organization.

Incorporate Video Communication:

Facilitate Virtual Interaction: Use video communication tools to facilitate interactions with family members and friends, especially if in-person visits are not possible.

Enhance Connectivity: Ensure that technology is user-friendly and accessible for the individual. Provide guidance and support for using technological aids.

10. Build a Supportive Environment

Create a Positive Atmosphere:

Foster a Supportive Environment: Create a positive and supportive communication environment by promoting respect, empathy, and understanding.

Encourage Open Dialogue: Encourage open dialogue and expression of feelings within the caregiving environment. Promote a culture of respect and support.

Educate and Train Caregivers:

Provide Training: Offer training and education for caregivers on effective communication strategies and techniques. Equip caregivers with the skills and knowledge to enhance interactions.

Share Best Practices: Share best practices and strategies for effective communication with all caregivers involved in the individual's care.

Effective communication in dementia care requires patience, adaptability, and understanding. By implementing these strategies, caregivers can improve interactions, support the individual's needs, and foster a positive and supportive caregiving environment.

Handling Challenging Behaviors in Dementia Care

Dealing with challenging behaviors in dementia care requires patience, empathy, and strategic approaches to manage situations effectively and maintain the well-being of both the individual with dementia and their caregivers. Here's a comprehensive guide on handling challenging behaviors:

1. Understanding the Underlying Causes

Identify Triggers:

Observe Patterns: Pay attention to patterns or triggers that lead to challenging behaviors. Common triggers include changes in routine, environmental factors, or unmet needs.

Assess Environmental Factors: Evaluate the environment for potential sources of stress or discomfort, such as noise, clutter, or uncomfortable temperatures.

Consider Medical Issues:

Check for Pain or Discomfort: Determine if the individual is experiencing pain, discomfort, or other medical issues that might be contributing to their behavior.

Review Medication Effects: Assess if any medications might be causing side effects or contributing to behavioral changes. Consult with healthcare providers for adjustments if needed.

Evaluate Emotional Needs:

Assess Emotional State: Consider if the individual is experiencing feelings of anxiety, frustration, or sadness that may be influencing their behavior.

Provide Emotional Support: Offer emotional support and reassurance to address underlying feelings and provide comfort.

2. Implementing De-Escalation Techniques

Remain Calm and Composed:

Use a Soothing Tone: Speak in a calm and soothing tone to help de-escalate the situation. Avoid raising your voice or appearing frustrated.

Practice Controlled Breathing: Use controlled breathing techniques to stay calm and manage your own stress during challenging moments.

Redirect Attention:

Change Focus: Gently redirect the individual's attention to a different activity or topic. For example, if they are agitated about an activity, suggest a calming or engaging alternative.

Introduce Distractions: Offer distractions such as a favorite object, music, or a simple game to shift their focus and reduce agitation.

Use Positive Reinforcement:

Acknowledge Positive Behavior: Recognize and praise any positive behavior or cooperation. Reinforce desired behaviors with encouragement and positive reinforcement.

Offer Incentives: Provide small rewards or incentives for participating in activities or following instructions. Positive reinforcement can help motivate and reduce challenging behaviors.

3. Adapting Communication Approaches

Simplify Instructions:

Use Clear Language: Communicate using clear, simple language and avoid complex instructions. Break tasks into manageable steps and provide one instruction at a time.

Use Visual Aids: Incorporate visual aids or demonstrations to support verbal instructions and enhance understanding.

Practice Empathetic Listening:

Acknowledge Feelings: Listen actively and acknowledge the individual's feelings and concerns. Show empathy and validate their emotions to build trust and understanding.

Respond with Compassion: Respond to their concerns with compassion and reassurance. Avoid arguing or dismissing their feelings.

Adjust Communication Style:

Modify Your Approach: Adjust your communication style based on the individual's cognitive abilities and preferences. Use gestures, facial expressions, and visual cues to support verbal communication.

4. Creating a Supportive Environment

Ensure a Calm Atmosphere:

Minimize Distractions: Reduce background noise and environmental distractions to create a calm and focused environment.

Adjust Lighting: Use appropriate lighting to enhance visibility and reduce shadows that may cause confusion or anxiety.

Establish Consistent Routines:

Maintain Regular Schedules: Establish and maintain consistent daily routines to provide structure and predictability. Consistent routines can help reduce anxiety and confusion.

Offer Familiar Activities: Incorporate familiar activities and routines to create a sense of security and comfort.

Personalize the Environment:

Use Familiar Objects: Surround the individual with familiar objects and personal items to create a sense of belonging and stability.

Adapt the Space: Modify the living space to meet the individual's needs and preferences, including safety features and comfort adjustments.

5. Managing Specific Challenging Behaviors

Aggression or Agitation:

Stay Safe: Ensure the safety of both the individual and caregivers. If necessary, remove yourself from the situation and seek assistance.

Identify Triggers: Determine the cause of aggression or agitation and address any underlying issues. Use calming techniques and avoid confrontational responses.

Wandering:

Implement Safety Measures: Use safety measures such as alarms, secure doors, or tracking devices to prevent wandering and ensure the individual's safety.

Redirect Attention: Redirect the individual's attention to engaging activities or offer a structured activity to reduce wandering tendencies.

Repetitive Questions or Behaviors:

Provide Reassurance: Offer reassurance and respond to repetitive questions with consistent, calm answers. Avoid showing frustration or irritation.

Introduce New Activities: Provide engaging activities or distractions to redirect focus and reduce repetitive behaviors.

6. Encouraging Positive Engagement

Promote Meaningful Activities:

Identify Interests: Engage the individual in activities that align with their interests and abilities. Meaningful activities can promote positive behavior and engagement.

Incorporate Hobbies: Include hobbies and favorite pastimes in daily routines to maintain a sense of purpose and enjoyment.

Foster Social Interaction:

Encourage Socialization: Facilitate opportunities for social interaction with family, friends, or community groups. Social engagement can improve mood and reduce challenging behaviors.

Create Social Opportunities: Plan social activities or outings that align with the individual's preferences and comfort level.

Provide a Sense of Accomplishment:

Offer Tasks: Provide simple tasks or activities that the individual can complete successfully. A sense of accomplishment can boost self-esteem and reduce frustration.

Celebrate Achievements: Recognize and celebrate small achievements and positive behavior to reinforce a sense of accomplishment and motivation.

Handling challenging behaviors in dementia care requires a combination of empathy, strategic approaches, and ongoing support. By implementing these strategies, caregivers can effectively manage behaviors, improve quality of life, and provide compassionate care.

Providing Emotional Support in Dementia Care

Providing emotional support is crucial in dementia care, as individuals with dementia often face significant emotional challenges, including feelings of confusion, frustration, and isolation. Offering compassionate and effective emotional support helps enhance their quality of life and fosters a positive caregiving environment. Here's a comprehensive guide to providing emotional support in dementia care:

1. Recognizing Emotional Needs

Observe Emotional States:

Monitor Mood Changes: Pay close attention to mood swings, signs of distress, or changes in behavior that may indicate emotional needs.

Identify Triggers: Identify events, interactions, or environmental factors that may trigger emotional responses or distress.

Validate Feelings:

Acknowledge Emotions: Validate the individual's emotions and feelings by acknowledging their experiences and providing reassurance.

Avoid Dismissing Concerns: Avoid dismissing or minimizing their concerns. Instead, show empathy and understanding.

Assess Needs Regularly:

Conduct Check-ins: Regularly check in with the individual to assess their emotional well-being and address any emerging needs.

Adapt to Changes: Be flexible and adapt to changes in emotional needs as the individual's condition progresses.

2. Offering Reassurance and Comfort

Provide Verbal Reassurance:

Use Soothing Words: Speak in a calming and reassuring manner to provide comfort. Use phrases that offer support and understanding.

Encourage Positive Thoughts: Offer encouragement and positive reinforcement to help the individual feel more secure and supported.

Offer Physical Comfort:

Use Gentle Touch: Provide physical comfort through gentle touch, such as holding hands or offering a hug, if appropriate and comforting.

Create a Comfortable Environment: Ensure that the physical environment is comfortable and conducive to relaxation, such as adjusting lighting and temperature.

Be Present and Attentive:

Give Full Attention: Provide undivided attention during interactions to show that you are fully present and engaged.

Practice Active Listening: Listen attentively to the individual's concerns and feelings, and respond with empathy and understanding.

3. Supporting Coping Strategies

Encourage Expression:

Promote Communication: Encourage the individual to express their feelings and thoughts through verbal communication, writing, or other forms of expression.

Provide Opportunities for Expression: Offer activities such as art, music, or journaling that allow the individual to express themselves creatively.

Develop Coping Techniques:

Introduce Relaxation Methods: Teach and encourage relaxation techniques, such as deep breathing exercises, mindfulness, or gentle stretching, to manage stress and anxiety.

Offer Distractions: Provide engaging activities or distractions to help redirect focus and alleviate distress.

Support Daily Routines:

Maintain Structure: Maintain a consistent daily routine to provide a sense of stability and predictability, which can help reduce anxiety.

Incorporate Familiar Activities: Include familiar activities and hobbies in daily routines to promote a sense of normalcy and enjoyment.

4. Building a Positive Relationship

Foster Trust and Respect:

Build Trust: Establish and maintain trust by being reliable, consistent, and respectful in all interactions.

Show Respect: Respect the individual's dignity, autonomy, and personal preferences in all aspects of care.

Engage in Meaningful Activities:

Find Enjoyable Activities: Identify and engage in activities that the individual enjoys and finds meaningful. Participation in enjoyable activities can boost mood and emotional well-being.

Promote Social Interaction: Facilitate social interactions with family, friends, or community groups to provide opportunities for connection and support.

Celebrate Achievements:

Recognize Accomplishments: Celebrate and acknowledge the individual's achievements and positive behavior, no matter how small.

Offer Praise: Provide praise and encouragement to reinforce positive behavior and build self-esteem.

5. Addressing Emotional Distress

Respond to Anxiety and Fear:

Provide Reassurance: Offer reassurance and comfort to address feelings of anxiety and fear. Use calming techniques and provide a sense of safety.

Identify and Address Sources of Fear: Identify potential sources of fear or anxiety and address them to reduce distress.

Manage Frustration and Anger:

Use De-Escalation Techniques: Implement de-escalation techniques, such as redirecting attention or offering calming distractions, to manage frustration and anger.

Validate Feelings: Acknowledge and validate the individual's feelings of frustration or anger, and provide support and understanding.

Support Coping with Loss:

Acknowledge Loss: Recognize and validate any feelings of loss or grief related to changes in cognitive abilities, independence, or personal identity.

Offer Support and Understanding: Provide support and understanding as the individual copes with loss and adjusts to changes in their condition.

6. Engaging in Collaborative Care

Involve the Individual:

Include in Decision-Making: Involve the individual in decisions related to their care and daily activities to promote a sense of control and autonomy.

Respect Preferences: Respect the individual's preferences and choices in care decisions and activities.

Collaborate with Family:

Communicate with Family Members: Maintain open communication with family members to ensure a collaborative approach to care and emotional support.

Share Insights and Strategies: Share insights and strategies for providing emotional support with family members to promote consistency and understanding.

Work with Professionals:

Seek Professional Guidance: Consult with healthcare professionals, such as psychologists or counselors, for additional support and guidance in managing emotional challenges.

Providing emotional support in dementia care involves understanding the individual's emotional needs, offering reassurance and comfort, and creating a supportive environment. By implementing these strategies, caregivers can enhance the individual's emotional well-being and contribute to a positive and compassionate caregiving experience.

SELF-CARE FOR CAREGIVERS

Self-care is essential for caregivers to maintain their own health and well-being while providing support to others. Caring for someone with dementia can be demanding and emotionally taxing, making it crucial for caregivers to prioritize their own needs to sustain effective caregiving.

Self-care for caregivers is essential for maintaining health, managing stress, and providing effective care. By implementing these strategies, caregivers can enhance their own well-being, prevent burnout, and continue to provide compassionate and effective support to those in their care.

Managing Stress and Burnout

Managing stress and burnout is crucial for caregivers to maintain their well-being and provide effective care. Caregiving can be a demanding role, often leading to significant emotional and physical stress. Addressing these challenges proactively can prevent burnout and support a healthier caregiving experience. Here's a comprehensive guide on managing stress and burnout:

1. Recognizing Stress and Burnout

Identify Symptoms:

Physical Symptoms: Recognize physical signs of stress and burnout, such as chronic fatigue, headaches, sleep disturbances, and gastrointestinal issues.

Emotional Symptoms: Be aware of emotional symptoms like anxiety, depression, irritability, and feelings of overwhelm or helplessness.

Behavioral Symptoms: Notice changes in behavior, such as withdrawal from social activities, increased irritability, and difficulty concentrating.

Acknowledge Your Limits:

Understand Personal Boundaries: Recognize that everyone has limits and it is important to acknowledge and accept them to prevent excessive strain.

Set Realistic Expectations: Set realistic expectations for yourself and caregiving responsibilities to avoid overloading yourself.

Assess Caregiving Demands:

Evaluate Workload: Regularly assess the demands and responsibilities of caregiving to identify areas where adjustments or support may be needed.

Identify Stressors: Identify specific stressors related to caregiving and develop strategies to address them.

2. Implementing Stress Reduction Techniques

Practice Relaxation Techniques:

Deep Breathing: Engage in deep breathing exercises to reduce stress and promote relaxation. Inhale slowly through the nose, hold, and exhale through the mouth.

Progressive Muscle Relaxation: Use progressive muscle relaxation techniques to relieve physical tension by systematically tensing and relaxing muscle groups.

Incorporate Mindfulness and Meditation:

Mindfulness: Practice mindfulness by focusing on the present moment and accepting thoughts and feelings without judgment. Techniques include mindful breathing and body scans.

Meditation: Engage in meditation practices to calm the mind and reduce stress. Options include guided meditation, mantra meditation, and loving-kindness meditation.

Engage in Physical Activity:

Exercise Regularly: Incorporate regular physical activity, such as walking, jogging, or yoga, to improve mood and reduce stress. Choose activities that you enjoy.

Practice Stretching: Perform stretching exercises to relieve physical tension and promote relaxation.

3. Building a Support System

Connect with Support Groups:

Join Caregiver Support Groups: Participate in caregiver support groups to share experiences, gain insights, and receive emotional support from others in similar situations.

Utilize Online Forums: Engage with online forums and communities to connect with other caregivers and access resources and advice.

Seek Professional Counseling:

Consult a Therapist: Consider consulting a mental health professional, such as a therapist or counselor, to address emotional challenges and develop coping strategies.

Participate in Counseling Sessions: Attend individual or group counseling sessions to receive support and guidance.

Engage with Family and Friends:

Share Responsibilities: Communicate with family and friends about caregiving responsibilities and seek their assistance or support.

Request Help: Don't hesitate to ask for help from loved ones to share caregiving duties and provide emotional support.

4. Prioritizing Self-Care

Establish a Self-Care Routine:

Schedule Personal Time: Allocate regular time for self-care activities, such as hobbies, relaxation, and personal interests.

Practice Self-Care Activities: Engage in self-care activities that promote well-being, such as reading, taking baths, or enjoying nature.

Set Boundaries:

Define Limits: Set clear boundaries between caregiving responsibilities and personal time to maintain balance and avoid overcommitment.

Communicate Needs: Communicate your needs and boundaries to others involved in caregiving to ensure a supportive environment.

Seek Respite Care:

Utilize Respite Services: Explore respite care options to provide temporary relief from caregiving duties and allow yourself time to rest and recharge.

Arrange for Temporary Care: Arrange for temporary care from professional caregivers or care facilities to take breaks and manage stress.

5. Managing Caregiver Burnout

Recognize Early Signs:

Monitor Burnout Indicators: Be vigilant for early signs of burnout, such as chronic exhaustion, increased irritability, and decreased motivation.

Address Issues Promptly: Address signs of burnout early by seeking support and making necessary adjustments to caregiving responsibilities.

Adjust Caregiving Duties:

Delegate Tasks: Delegate caregiving tasks to others, such as family members or professional caregivers, to reduce the burden and alleviate stress.

Reevaluate Responsibilities: Reevaluate and adjust caregiving responsibilities as needed to better manage stress and prevent burnout.

Seek Professional Support:

Consult with Professionals: Seek guidance from healthcare professionals, such as counselors or social workers, to address burnout and develop effective coping strategies.

Access Support Services: Utilize available support services and resources designed to assist caregivers in managing stress and burnout.

6. Creating a Balanced Lifestyle

Maintain a Healthy Work-Life Balance:

Balance Caregiving and Personal Life: Strive to balance caregiving responsibilities with personal time and activities to ensure a well-rounded lifestyle.

Set Priorities: Prioritize personal well-being and self-care alongside caregiving duties to maintain overall health and satisfaction.

Engage in Leisure Activities:

Pursue Enjoyable Hobbies: Engage in leisure activities and hobbies that bring joy and relaxation, providing a break from caregiving responsibilities.

Plan Regular Outings: Schedule regular outings or events that you enjoy to enhance your quality of life and reduce stress.

Focus on Positive Experiences:

Celebrate Achievements: Celebrate personal and caregiving achievements to foster a sense of accomplishment and boost morale.

Managing stress and burnout requires a proactive and multifaceted approach. By implementing these strategies, caregivers can effectively manage stress, prevent burnout, and maintain their well-being while providing compassionate care.

Seeking Support and Respite

Caregiving can be demanding, and seeking support and respite is crucial for maintaining your well-being and effectiveness as a caregiver. Respite care provides temporary relief from caregiving duties, while seeking support helps manage the emotional and practical challenges of caregiving. Here's a comprehensive guide on seeking support and respite:

1. Understanding the Need for Respite

Recognize the Importance:

Prevent Burnout: Understand that regular breaks are essential to prevent caregiver burnout and maintain overall health.

Recharge and Rejuvenate: Acknowledge that taking time away from caregiving responsibilities allows you to recharge and return with renewed energy and perspective.

Assess Your Needs:

Evaluate Caregiving Demands: Assess the intensity and duration of your caregiving duties to determine the need for respite.

Identify Personal Limitations: Recognize your personal limitations and understand that seeking respite is a proactive step toward self-care.

Determine Respite Options:

Explore Available Services: Research various respite care options, such as in-home respite services, adult day programs, or short-term care facilities.

Consider Your Preferences: Choose respite options that align with your preferences and the needs of the person you are caring for.

2. Exploring Respite Care Options

In-Home Respite Services:

Hire Professional Caregivers: Engage professional caregivers or respite providers who can offer temporary care in your home, allowing you to take a break.

Utilize Home Health Aides: Employ home health aides to assist with daily activities and provide care while you are away.

Adult Day Programs:

Attend Day Centers: Explore adult day centers that offer structured activities and care during the day, providing relief for caregivers.

Participate in Social Programs: Utilize programs that offer socialization, therapy, and recreational activities for individuals with dementia.

Short-Term Care Facilities:

Consider Respite Stays: Look into short-term stays at care facilities or assisted living communities that provide temporary care and support.

Assess Facility Options: Evaluate different facilities based on their services, environment, and compatibility with the individual's needs.

3. Seeking Emotional and Practical Support

Connect with Support Groups:

Join Caregiver Support Groups: Participate in caregiver support groups to share experiences, receive emotional support, and gain practical advice.

Engage in Online Communities: Join online forums or social media groups for caregivers to connect with others and access resources.

Consult Professional Counselors:

Seek Therapy or Counseling: Consider professional counseling or therapy to address emotional challenges, stress, and caregiver burnout.

Access Support Services: Utilize mental health services designed for caregivers to receive personalized support and guidance.

Leverage Community Resources:

Utilize Local Services: Explore community resources, such as nonprofit organizations and local agencies, that offer support and assistance for caregivers.

Participate in Workshops: Attend workshops or educational programs focused on caregiving skills, stress management, and self-care.

4. Communicating Your Needs

Discuss Respite with Family:

Coordinate with Family Members: Communicate your need for respite to family members and discuss how they can assist with caregiving duties.

Seek Shared Responsibility: Collaborate with family members to share caregiving responsibilities and provide support.

Request Support from Friends:

Reach Out for Assistance: Ask friends for help with caregiving tasks or to provide companionship and support during breaks.

Build a Support Network: Develop a network of friends who can offer practical assistance and emotional support.

Communicate with Healthcare Providers:

Discuss Care Needs: Talk to healthcare providers about your respite needs and seek recommendations for respite services or support.

Address Concerns: Share any concerns or challenges you are facing with healthcare providers to receive appropriate guidance and support.

5. Planning and Organizing Respite Care

Create a Respite Plan:

Develop a Schedule: Establish a respite schedule that includes regular breaks and planned time off to ensure consistent self-care.

Plan Ahead: Make arrangements for respite care in advance to ensure availability and a smooth transition.

Prepare for Respite Care:

Provide Detailed Instructions: Prepare detailed instructions and information for respite caregivers to ensure continuity of care.

Ensure Comfort: Make sure the individual's needs and preferences are communicated to the respite provider to ensure comfort and satisfaction.

Monitor Respite Experiences:

Evaluate Effectiveness: Monitor and assess the effectiveness of respite care to ensure it meets your needs and those of the person you are caring for.

Adjust as Needed: Make adjustments to the respite plan based on feedback and experiences to optimize the respite process.

6. Managing Respite Transitions

Smooth Transitions:

Prepare the Individual: Prepare the person you are caring for for the transition to respite care by explaining the process and addressing any concerns.

Ensure Continuity: Maintain continuity of care by providing clear instructions and maintaining communication with respite providers.

Evaluate Respite Care:

Assess Quality of Care: Evaluate the quality of care provided during respite to ensure it meets your standards and expectations.

Provide Feedback: Offer feedback to respite providers to improve the quality of care and address any issues.

Reflect and Adjust:

Reflect on Experiences: Reflect on your experiences with respite care to identify what worked well and what could be improved.

Adjust Plans: Make necessary adjustments to your respite care plans based on your reflections and experiences.

7. Utilizing Professional Respite Services

Research Professional Providers:

Explore Options: Research and compare professional respite care providers to find those that best meet your needs and preferences.

Check Credentials: Verify the credentials and qualifications of professional caregivers and respite service providers.

Evaluate Service Quality:

Review Feedback: Check reviews and feedback from other caregivers who have used the services to assess the quality and reliability of providers.

Interview Providers: Conduct interviews with potential providers to discuss their services, experience, and approach to care.

Understand Costs and Coverage:

Review Pricing: Understand the costs associated with professional respite services and determine how they fit into your budget.

Check Insurance Coverage: Verify if your insurance covers respite care services and explore financial assistance options if needed.

8. Addressing Caregiver Needs

Prioritize Your Well-Being:

Focus on Self-Care: Prioritize your own physical, emotional, and mental well-being by integrating self-care practices into your routine.

Seek Personal Fulfillment: Engage in activities that bring you joy and fulfillment outside of caregiving responsibilities.

Maintain Balance:

Balance Responsibilities: Strive to balance caregiving duties with personal interests and responsibilities to avoid becoming overwhelmed.

Set Boundaries: Establish clear boundaries between caregiving and personal time to maintain a healthy work-life balance.

Access Support Resources:

Utilize Available Resources: Take advantage of support resources, such as educational materials, counseling services, and support groups.

Explore New Options: Continuously explore new support options and resources to enhance your caregiving experience.

9. Building a Resilient Support Network

Develop Connections:

Network with Other Caregivers: Connect with other caregivers to share experiences, exchange tips, and provide mutual support.

Engage with Community Organizations: Participate in community organizations and programs that offer support and resources for caregivers.

Foster Positive Relationships:

Cultivate Relationships: Build and maintain positive relationships with family, friends, and support network members.

Encourage Open Communication: Foster open communication with your support network to address needs and concerns effectively.

Strengthen Support Systems:

Expand Your Network: Expand your support network by seeking out additional resources and connections that can provide assistance and encouragement.

Leverage Community Resources: Utilize community resources and organizations to strengthen your support system and enhance caregiving support.

10. Continuing Self-Education and Growth

Stay Informed:

Educate Yourself: Stay informed about caregiving practices, stress management techniques, and available support resources.

Attend Workshops and Seminars: Participate in workshops, seminars, and training sessions to enhance your caregiving skills and knowledge.

Seek Personal Development:

Pursue Personal Growth: Engage in personal development activities, such as continuing education, hobbies, or volunteering, to enhance your well-being and resilience.

Reflect on Growth: Regularly reflect on your personal growth and achievements as a caregiver to build confidence and motivation.

Embrace Adaptability:

Adapt to Change: Be flexible and adaptable in your caregiving role, adjusting to changes in the individual's needs and your own circumstances.

Explore New Resources: Continuously explore new resources and strategies to improve your caregiving experience and personal well-being.

Seeking support and respite is essential for managing the demands of caregiving and maintaining your well-being. By utilizing available resources, communicating your needs, and prioritizing self-care, you can effectively manage stress and prevent burnout, ensuring a healthier and more fulfilling caregiving experience.

Maintaining Personal Health

Maintaining personal health is vital for caregivers to sustain their well-being and provide effective care. Caregiving often involves significant emotional and physical demands, making it essential to prioritize your own health and wellness. To maintain personal health while caregiving:

1. Prioritizing Physical Health

Regular Exercise:

Incorporate Physical Activity: Engage in regular exercise such as walking, jogging, swimming, or strength training to boost energy levels, reduce stress, and improve overall fitness.

Find Enjoyable Activities: Choose physical activities that you enjoy to make exercise a more pleasant and sustainable part of your routine.

Healthy Eating:

Balanced Diet: Consume a balanced diet rich in fruits, vegetables, whole grains, lean proteins, and healthy fats to maintain energy levels and support overall health.

Stay Hydrated: Drink plenty of water throughout the day to stay hydrated and support bodily functions.

Adequate Sleep:

Establish a Sleep Routine: Create a consistent sleep routine by going to bed and waking up at the same time each day to ensure restorative rest.

Create a Sleep-Friendly Environment: Optimize your sleep environment by keeping it dark, quiet, and cool to promote better sleep quality.

2. Managing Stress Effectively

Stress Reduction Techniques:

Practice Relaxation Methods: Use relaxation techniques such as deep breathing, progressive muscle relaxation, or guided imagery to manage stress and promote relaxation.

Engage in Mindfulness: Incorporate mindfulness practices, such as meditation or mindful breathing, to stay present and reduce anxiety.

Time Management:

Organize Your Schedule: Plan and prioritize tasks to manage your time effectively and reduce feelings of being overwhelmed.

Set Realistic Goals: Set achievable goals and break tasks into smaller, manageable steps to reduce stress and increase productivity.

Seek Emotional Support:

Connect with Support Networks: Engage with support groups, friends, or family members to share your experiences and receive emotional support.

Consult a Therapist: Consider professional counseling or therapy to address emotional challenges and develop coping strategies.

3. Maintaining Mental Health

Mental Stimulation:

Engage in Cognitive Activities: Stimulate your mind through activities such as reading, puzzles, or learning new skills to keep your cognitive functions active.

Pursue Hobbies and Interests: Make time for hobbies and interests that bring you joy and satisfaction to support mental well-being.

Emotional Expression:

Express Feelings: Allow yourself to express emotions and feelings, whether through talking, writing, or creative outlets, to manage stress and emotional strain.

Practice Self-Compassion: Be kind to yourself and recognize that it's okay to experience and express a range of emotions.

Professional Help:

Seek Counseling: If you're experiencing persistent mental health challenges, seek help from a mental health professional for guidance and support.

Explore Therapy Options: Consider different types of therapy, such as cognitive-behavioral therapy (CBT) or psychotherapy, to address mental health concerns.

4. Ensuring Regular Health Check-Ups

Schedule Routine Appointments:

Visit Healthcare Providers: Schedule regular check-ups with your primary care physician, dentist, and other healthcare providers to monitor and maintain your health.

Keep Up with Screenings: Stay up-to-date with recommended health screenings and preventive measures based on your age, gender, and medical history.

Monitor Health Conditions:

Manage Chronic Conditions: If you have any chronic health conditions, work with your healthcare provider to manage and monitor them effectively.

Track Symptoms: Keep track of any symptoms or health changes and report them to your healthcare provider promptly.

Adhere to Medical Advice:

Follow Treatment Plans: Adhere to prescribed treatments, medications, and lifestyle modifications recommended by your healthcare provider.

Seek Second Opinions: If needed, seek second opinions or consult specialists to ensure comprehensive and accurate health care.

5. Building a Supportive Environment

Create a Support System:

Develop Connections: Build relationships with family, friends, and support networks to create a reliable support system for emotional and practical assistance.

Seek Professional Support: Utilize professional support services, such as caregivers, counselors, or social workers, to assist with caregiving and personal needs.

Establish Boundaries:

Set Limits: Establish clear boundaries between caregiving responsibilities and personal time to maintain balance and avoid caregiver fatigue.

Communicate Needs: Clearly communicate your needs and limits to others involved in caregiving to ensure a supportive and understanding environment.

Foster a Positive Environment:

Create a Relaxing Space: Design a comfortable and relaxing environment at home where you can unwind and recharge.

Promote Positivity: Focus on positive aspects of caregiving and celebrate successes to maintain a hopeful and resilient outlook.

6. Engaging in Self-Care Practices

Prioritize Personal Time:

Schedule Self-Care: Allocate regular time for self-care activities, such as relaxation, hobbies, or personal interests, to support your well-being.

Set Aside Time for Yourself: Make time for activities that bring you joy and relaxation, and prioritize self-care in your daily routine.

Practice Relaxation:

Use Relaxation Techniques: Engage in activities that promote relaxation, such as reading, taking baths, or practicing mindfulness.

Explore Stress-Relief Options: Experiment with different stress-relief techniques, such as yoga, tai chi, or aromatherapy, to find what works best for you.

Seek Enjoyable Activities:

Participate in Hobbies: Engage in hobbies or activities that bring you pleasure and help you unwind from caregiving duties.

Explore New Interests: Try new activities or interests to keep your routine fresh and enjoyable.

7. Balancing Caregiving and Personal Life

Manage Time Wisely:

Create a Balanced Schedule: Develop a balanced schedule that includes time for caregiving, personal activities, and relaxation.

Delegate Tasks: Share caregiving responsibilities with others when possible to reduce your workload and prevent burnout.

Set Boundaries:

Define Personal Time: Set clear boundaries between caregiving and personal time to maintain a healthy balance and avoid overcommitment.

Communicate Limits: Communicate your boundaries and needs to family members and other caregivers to ensure mutual understanding.

Foster Personal Interests:

Pursue Personal Goals: Set and work towards personal goals and interests to maintain a sense of fulfillment and purpose outside of caregiving.

Enjoy Social Activities: Make time for social activities and relationships to maintain connections and support.

8. Addressing Financial Well-Being

Manage Finances:

Budget Effectively: Create and stick to a budget that accounts for caregiving expenses and personal financial needs.

Explore Financial Assistance: Research and apply for financial assistance programs or benefits available for caregivers.

Plan for Future Needs:

Save for Emergencies: Build an emergency fund to cover unexpected expenses and provide financial stability.

Review Insurance Coverage: Evaluate your insurance coverage and ensure it meets your needs and those of the person you are caring for.

Seek Financial Advice:

Consult Financial Advisors: Work with financial advisors to develop a plan for managing caregiving expenses and planning for future financial needs.

Explore Financial Resources: Utilize resources and programs designed to support caregivers financially.

9. Engaging in Regular Reflection

Assess Well-Being:

Reflect on Personal Health: Regularly assess your physical, mental, and emotional well-being to identify areas that need attention or improvement.

Adjust Self-Care Practices: Make adjustments to your self-care practices based on your reflections and changing needs.

Evaluate Caregiving Impact:

Review Caregiving Role: Reflect on how caregiving is impacting your health and well-being and make necessary adjustments to manage stress and balance responsibilities.

Seek Feedback: Seek feedback from trusted individuals to gain insights into how you can improve your self-care and overall health.

Celebrate Achievements:

Recognize Accomplishments: Acknowledge and celebrate your achievements and progress in managing caregiving and personal health.

Focus on Positive Outcomes: Maintain a positive outlook by focusing on the positive aspects of your caregiving journey and personal growth.

10. Continuing Personal Development

Pursue Growth Opportunities:

Engage in Learning: Pursue opportunities for personal growth and development, such as education, training, or skill-building activities.

Set Personal Goals: Establish and work towards personal goals that contribute to your overall well-being and satisfaction.

Explore New Interests:

Try New Activities: Explore new hobbies, interests, or activities to keep your life engaging and fulfilling.

Expand Horizons: Seek out new experiences and opportunities to enrich your life and personal growth.

Maintaining personal health is essential for effective caregiving and overall well-being. By prioritizing physical, mental, and emotional health, managing stress, seeking support, and engaging in self-care practices, you can sustain your health and provide compassionate and effective care.

FUTURE PLANNING AND END-OF-LIFE ISSUES

Future planning and addressing end-of-life issues are crucial aspects of caregiving, ensuring that both the individual's wishes and the caregiver's needs are considered. This section will guide you through key components of planning for the future and managing end-of-life issues effectively.

Planning for the Future

Planning for the future is essential in caregiving, ensuring that both the individual's needs and the caregiver's responsibilities are thoughtfully addressed. This proactive approach involves financial, legal, and personal preparations to manage future uncertainties and provide a structured framework for ongoing care. Here's a comprehensive guide on planning for the future:

1. Legal and Financial Preparation

Advanced Directives and Legal Documents:

Living Wills: Outline preferences for medical treatment if the individual becomes incapacitated.

Health Care Proxy: Designate a trusted person to make healthcare decisions on the individual's behalf.

Power of Attorney: Appoint someone to manage financial and legal matters.

Wills and Trusts: Create or update a will and consider establishing trusts to manage and distribute assets according to the individual's wishes.

Financial Planning:

Cost Estimation: Assess potential future costs for medical care, daily living expenses, and long-term care.

Budget Development: Create a detailed budget to manage current and projected expenses, considering sources of income and savings.

Long-Term Care Insurance: Explore and purchase long-term care insurance to help cover future care costs.

Public Benefits:

Social Security: Determine eligibility for benefits and explore options for disability or survivor benefits.

Medicare and Medicaid: Investigate eligibility and coverage options for Medicare and Medicaid to support healthcare needs.

2. Care Planning

Developing a Care Plan:

Comprehensive Assessment: Conduct a thorough assessment of current and future care needs, including medical, emotional, and personal support.

Care Goals: Set clear goals for care, considering the individual's preferences and needs.

Action Plan: Develop a detailed action plan to address care requirements, including medical treatments, daily living assistance, and special needs.

Coordinating Care:

Healthcare Providers: Establish and maintain communication with healthcare providers to ensure coordinated care.

Care Team: Assemble a care team that includes family members, professional caregivers, and other support resources.

Regular Reviews: Periodically review and update the care plan to reflect changes in health status and care needs.

3. Emergency Planning

Contingency Plans:

Emergency Contacts: Maintain an updated list of emergency contacts, including healthcare providers, family members, and legal representatives.

Emergency Procedures: Develop and document emergency procedures for medical crises, sudden changes in health, and other urgent situations.

Preparedness Kits:

Health Information: Keep a preparedness kit with essential health information, including medical records, medications, and care instructions.

Emergency Supplies: Stock necessary supplies, such as medications, first-aid items, and contact information for emergency services.

4. Personal and Lifestyle Considerations

Daily Living Arrangements:

Home Modifications: Plan for any necessary home modifications to accommodate future care needs, such as accessibility improvements and safety features.

Living Arrangements: Consider future living arrangements, including options for in-home care, assisted living, or nursing facilities.

Lifestyle Preferences:

Activity and Engagement: Plan for activities and social engagements that align with the individual's interests and preferences.

Quality of Life: Ensure that future planning addresses factors that contribute to a high quality of life, including comfort, enjoyment, and personal fulfillment.

5. Legal and Financial Documents

Document Storage:

Secure Location: Store important legal and financial documents in a secure and accessible location, such as a safe or secure digital storage.

Access for Key Individuals: Ensure that key individuals, such as family members and legal representatives, have access to necessary documents.

Review and Update:

Regular Updates: Periodically review and update legal and financial documents to reflect any changes in personal circumstances, laws, or regulations.

Professional Advice: Consult with legal and financial professionals to ensure that documents are current and legally valid.

6. Health and Wellness Planning

Medical Care:

Health Monitoring: Implement plans for regular health monitoring and medical check-ups to address changing health needs.

Specialist Care: Arrange for specialist care if needed and ensure that referrals and appointments are managed effectively.

Emotional and Psychological Support:

Counseling Services: Plan for access to counseling or therapy services to address emotional and psychological needs.

Support Networks: Develop a network of support, including friends, family, and support groups, to provide emotional and practical assistance.

7. End-of-Life Planning

Advance Planning:

End-of-Life Wishes: Document and communicate end-of-life preferences, including decisions about medical treatment, funeral arrangements, and other final wishes.

Funeral Pre-Arrangements: Consider making pre-arrangements for funeral and burial services to reduce the burden on family members.

Palliative and Hospice Care:

Care Options: Plan for palliative and hospice care to provide comfort and support during the end-of-life process.

Family Support: Ensure that family members are involved in discussions and decisions related to end-of-life care and support.

8. Educational and Training Resources

Learning Opportunities:

Training Programs: Enroll in training programs or workshops to enhance caregiving skills and knowledge.

Educational Materials: Utilize educational materials, such as books, online courses, and webinars, to stay informed about caregiving best practices.

Skill Development:

Skill Building: Focus on developing skills related to caregiving, such as managing medical needs, handling challenging behaviors, and providing emotional support.

Resource Utilization: Leverage available resources to improve caregiving effectiveness and ensure high-quality care.

9. Communication and Coordination

Family Discussions:

Open Communication: Foster open communication with family members about future plans, caregiving responsibilities, and personal preferences.

Coordination of Care: Coordinate caregiving efforts among family members to ensure consistency and effective support.

Care Team Meetings:

Regular Meetings: Schedule regular meetings with the care team to discuss updates, address concerns, and plan for ongoing care needs.

Collaborative Approach: Encourage collaboration and input from all members of the care team to ensure comprehensive and coordinated care.

10. Reflecting and Adapting

Reviewing Plans:

Regular Reflection: Periodically review and reflect on future planning efforts to ensure they continue to meet evolving needs and preferences.

Adaptation: Make necessary adjustments to plans based on changes in health, financial status, or personal circumstances.

Continuous Improvement:

Feedback and Learning: Seek feedback from family members and caregivers to improve planning and care strategies.

Ongoing Adaptation: Continuously adapt plans and strategies to address new challenges and opportunities for improvement.

Planning for the future requires careful consideration of legal, financial, and personal factors to ensure that both the individual's needs and the caregiver's responsibilities are effectively managed. By taking a proactive and organized approach, you can provide comprehensive support and create a structured framework for addressing future uncertainties.

Hospice and Palliative Care

Hospice and palliative care are specialized types of medical care designed to improve the quality of life for individuals facing serious, life-limiting illnesses. While they share some similarities, they serve distinct purposes and are tailored to different stages of illness and care needs. This guide outlines the principles, differences, and practical aspects of both types of care.

1. Understanding Hospice Care

Definition and Purpose:

Hospice Care: Focuses on providing comfort and support to individuals who are in the final stages of a terminal illness. The goal is to enhance the quality of life and ensure a peaceful end-of-life experience.

Approach: Emphasizes symptom management, pain relief, and emotional support rather than curative treatment. It is intended for individuals with a prognosis of six months or less to live if the illness follows its usual course.

Services Provided:

Medical Care: Includes pain and symptom management, coordinated by a team of healthcare professionals.

Emotional and Spiritual Support: Offers counseling and support for emotional and spiritual needs, both for the individual and their family.

Practical Support: Assists with daily living activities, such as personal care and homemaking, as needed.

Eligibility and Enrollment:

Eligibility Criteria: Typically requires a terminal diagnosis with a life expectancy of six months or less. Enrollment is based on the individual's and family's decision to focus on comfort rather than curative treatments.

Referral Process: Often initiated by a physician or healthcare provider, but families can also request hospice care.

2. Understanding Palliative Care

Definition and Purpose:

Palliative Care: Focuses on providing relief from symptoms, pain, and stress associated with serious illnesses, regardless of the stage of the disease. It is intended to improve quality of life for individuals and their families.

Approach: Can be provided alongside curative treatment or as the main approach when curative options are not feasible. It aims to address physical, emotional, and psychological distress.

Services Provided:

Symptom Management: Includes addressing symptoms such as pain, nausea, fatigue, and shortness of breath.

Supportive Care: Provides support for emotional, psychological, and social issues, helping individuals and families cope with the impact of illness.

Care Coordination: Coordinates care among various healthcare providers and specialists to ensure comprehensive support.

Eligibility and Enrollment:

Eligibility Criteria: Available to individuals at any stage of a serious illness, regardless of prognosis. Can be provided alongside other treatments aimed at curing or managing the illness.

Referral Process: Typically involves a referral from a healthcare provider, but can also be requested by the patient or family.

3. Key Differences Between Hospice and Palliative Care

Timing and Focus:

Hospice Care: Provided when curative treatments are no longer effective or desired, focusing solely on comfort and quality of life.

Palliative Care: Can be initiated at any stage of illness and is often provided alongside curative treatments, focusing on symptom relief and support.

Treatment Goals:

Hospice Care: Aims to provide comfort and dignity in the final stages of life, with an emphasis on easing pain and providing support.

Palliative Care: Aims to enhance quality of life through symptom management and supportive care, regardless of the stage of illness.

Care Settings:

Hospice Care: Can be provided at home, in hospice facilities, or in nursing homes. Care is often delivered by a team of healthcare professionals, including doctors, nurses, social workers, and volunteers.

Palliative Care: Typically provided in hospitals, outpatient clinics, or home settings. The care team may include physicians, nurses, social workers, and other specialists.

4. Implementing Hospice and Palliative Care

Assessing Needs:

Individual Assessment: Evaluate the individual's medical, emotional, and psychological needs to determine the appropriate type of care.

Family Involvement: Engage family members in discussions about care preferences and goals to ensure that the individual's wishes are respected.

Care Planning:

Customized Care Plans: Develop individualized care plans that address specific needs and preferences, incorporating input from healthcare providers and family members.

Regular Review: Regularly review and adjust care plans based on changes in the individual's condition and preferences.

Coordination of Care:

Multidisciplinary Team: Collaborate with a team of healthcare professionals, including doctors, nurses, social workers, and counselors, to provide comprehensive support.

Communication: Maintain open communication among all members of the care team, the individual, and their family to ensure coordinated and effective care.

5. Benefits and Challenges

Benefits:

Improved Quality of Life: Both hospice and palliative care focus on improving quality of life through symptom management and support.

Emotional and Psychological Support: Provides emotional, psychological, and spiritual support to individuals and their families.

Family Support: Offers support for family members, including counseling, respite care, and practical assistance.

Challenges:

Emotional Difficulties: Navigating end-of-life issues and serious illness can be emotionally challenging for individuals and families.

Care Coordination: Coordinating care among multiple providers and ensuring effective communication can be complex.

6. Accessing Hospice and Palliative Care

Finding Providers:

Healthcare Providers: Ask your primary care physician or specialist for recommendations on hospice and palliative care providers.

Referrals: Obtain referrals from hospitals, community health organizations, or local support groups.

Insurance and Coverage:

Insurance Plans: Check with your health insurance provider to understand coverage options for hospice and palliative care services.

Financial Assistance: Explore available financial assistance programs, including government benefits and charitable organizations, to help cover care costs.

7. Support for Families and Caregivers

Emotional Support:

Counseling: Access counseling services to help cope with the emotional impact of caregiving and end-of-life issues.

Support Groups: Join support groups to connect with others facing similar challenges and share experiences.

Practical Assistance:

Respite Care: Utilize respite care services to provide temporary relief for primary caregivers.

Training and Resources: Seek training and resources to enhance caregiving skills and manage care effectively.

8. Preparing for End-of-Life

Discussing Wishes:

Advance Directives: Ensure that advance directives and end-of-life wishes are documented and communicated to healthcare providers and family members.

Care Preferences: Discuss and document preferences for end-of-life care, including pain management, comfort measures, and final arrangements.

Making Arrangements:

Funeral Planning: Consider pre-arranging funeral services and discussing final wishes with family members.

Legal and Financial Planning: Address legal and financial matters, including wills, power of attorney, and estate planning.

9. Reflecting on Care

Evaluating Care:

Care Quality: Reflect on the quality of care provided and assess whether it met the individual's needs and preferences.

Feedback: Provide feedback to healthcare providers and care teams to improve future care practices and support.

Learning and Improvement:

Personal Growth: Reflect on the caregiving experience to gain insights and improve future caregiving approaches.

Resource Utilization: Use lessons learned to better utilize available resources and support services.

Community Organizations:

Local Services: Contact local community organizations and health services for additional support and resources related to hospice and palliative care.

National Organizations: Reach out to national organizations, such as the Hospice and Palliative Care Organization, for information and support.

Hospice and palliative care are vital components of managing serious illnesses and end-of-life care. By understanding the principles and practical aspects of these types of care, individuals and families can make informed decisions, enhance quality of life, and ensure compassionate support throughout the caregiving journey.

Coping with Loss and Grief

Coping with loss and grief is a profound and personal journey that involves navigating the emotional, psychological, and practical impacts of losing a loved one. Understanding the grieving process and finding effective ways to manage and support oneself during this challenging time is crucial for healing and recovery. Here's a comprehensive guide to help navigate this difficult experience:

1. Understanding Grief

Grief and Its Stages:

Stages of Grief: Commonly described by the Kubler-Ross model, which includes denial, anger, bargaining, depression, and acceptance. These stages are not linear and individuals may experience them in different orders or revisit stages.

Emotional Responses: Grief can manifest through a range of emotions, including sadness, anger, guilt, and confusion. These feelings are normal and part of the grieving process.

Types of Grief:

Normal Grief: The typical emotional response to loss, which may include a mix of sadness, anger, and relief. It usually diminishes over time as individuals adjust to the loss.

Complicated Grief: Persistent and intense grief that interferes with daily functioning. It may involve prolonged sadness, difficulty moving forward, or unresolved feelings about the loss.

Physical and Cognitive Impact:

Physical Symptoms: Grief can affect physical health, leading to symptoms such as fatigue, changes in appetite, and sleep disturbances.

Cognitive Effects: Difficulty concentrating, forgetfulness, and confusion are common cognitive responses to grief.

2. Coping Strategies

Emotional Expression:

Talking About Feelings: Expressing emotions through conversation with friends, family, or a counselor can help process grief.

Writing: Keeping a journal or writing letters to the deceased can provide an outlet for emotions and reflections.

Self-Care:

Healthy Habits: Maintain a balanced diet, regular exercise, and sufficient sleep to support physical and emotional well-being.

Relaxation Techniques: Practice mindfulness, meditation, or deep breathing exercises to manage stress and anxiety.

Seeking Professional Help:

Counseling: Engage with a therapist or grief counselor for professional support in managing complex or prolonged grief.

Support Groups: Join support groups for individuals experiencing similar losses to share experiences and receive comfort from others.

3. Supporting Others in Grief

Providing Comfort:

Listening: Offer a compassionate ear and allow individuals to share their feelings and memories without judgment.

Practical Help: Provide practical support, such as helping with daily tasks, meals, or childcare, to ease the burden during the grieving period.

Respecting Individual Needs:

Personal Space: Respect the need for solitude or personal space while also offering companionship and support when needed.

Customizing Support: Understand and respect the unique ways in which individuals grieve and offer support that aligns with their preferences.

4. Navigating Grief Milestones

Anniversaries and Holidays:

Acknowledging Dates: Recognize important dates, such as anniversaries and holidays, which may trigger intense emotions. Plan for these times by creating rituals or seeking support.

Creating New Traditions: Establish new traditions or ways to honor the memory of the deceased during special occasions.

Adjusting to Changes:

New Routines: Adapt to changes in daily routines and responsibilities that may arise due to the loss. Seek support in adjusting to these new roles.

Finding Meaning: Explore ways to find meaning or purpose following the loss, such as through personal growth, charitable activities, or memorializing the loved one.

5. Addressing Complex Grief Issues

Traumatic Loss:

Processing Trauma: Seek specialized support if the loss involves trauma, such as sudden or violent death, which can complicate the grieving process.

Professional Therapy: Engage in therapy focused on trauma and grief to address specific emotional and psychological challenges.

Family Dynamics:

Family Grieving Styles: Recognize and navigate differences in grieving styles among family members. Facilitate open communication and mutual support.

Conflict Resolution: Address and resolve conflicts that may arise within families due to differing grief responses or responsibilities.

6. Long-Term Healing

Personal Growth:

Self-Reflection: Engage in self-reflection and personal development to integrate the loss into one's life and find a new sense of purpose.

Continued Support: Continue seeking support as needed, recognizing that grief may persist or resurface at different times.

Building Resilience:

Strengths and Skills: Focus on building resilience by developing coping skills and drawing on personal strengths.

Community Involvement: Engage in community or social activities that provide a sense of connection and support.

Professional Organizations:

Grief Support Organizations: Connect with organizations specializing in grief support, such as The Hospice Foundation of America or the National Alliance for Grieving Children.

Local Services: Reach out to local mental health professionals and support services for personalized assistance.

8. Cultural and Religious Considerations

Cultural Practices:

Understanding Traditions: Respect and incorporate cultural or religious practices related to grieving and mourning, which may offer comfort and structure.

Community Rituals: Participate in community rituals or ceremonies that align with cultural or religious beliefs to honor the deceased.

Spiritual Support:

Spiritual Counseling: Seek support from spiritual leaders or counselors who can provide guidance and comfort based on spiritual or religious beliefs.

Faith-Based Practices: Engage in faith-based practices, such as prayer or meditation, to find solace and meaning.

9. Preparing for Grief's Impact

Anticipatory Grief:

Preparing Emotionally: If anticipating a loss, prepare emotionally by seeking support, discussing feelings, and creating meaningful memories with the loved one.

Care Planning: Plan for practical aspects of caregiving and end-of-life arrangements to ease the burden when the loss occurs.

Educational Preparation:

Grief Education: Educate oneself and family members about the grieving process to better understand and navigate the experience.

10. Finding Support

Community Connections:

Support Networks: Build and maintain connections with friends, family, and community organizations for ongoing support.

Volunteer Opportunities: Engage in volunteer opportunities or community activities that provide a sense of purpose and connection.

Coping with loss and grief is a deeply personal journey that requires time, patience, and support. By understanding the grieving process, utilizing effective coping strategies, and seeking appropriate resources, individuals can navigate their grief with compassion and resilience.

Made in United States
Troutdale, OR
09/01/2024

22496430R00080